# The
# Simply Vegan
## Cookbook

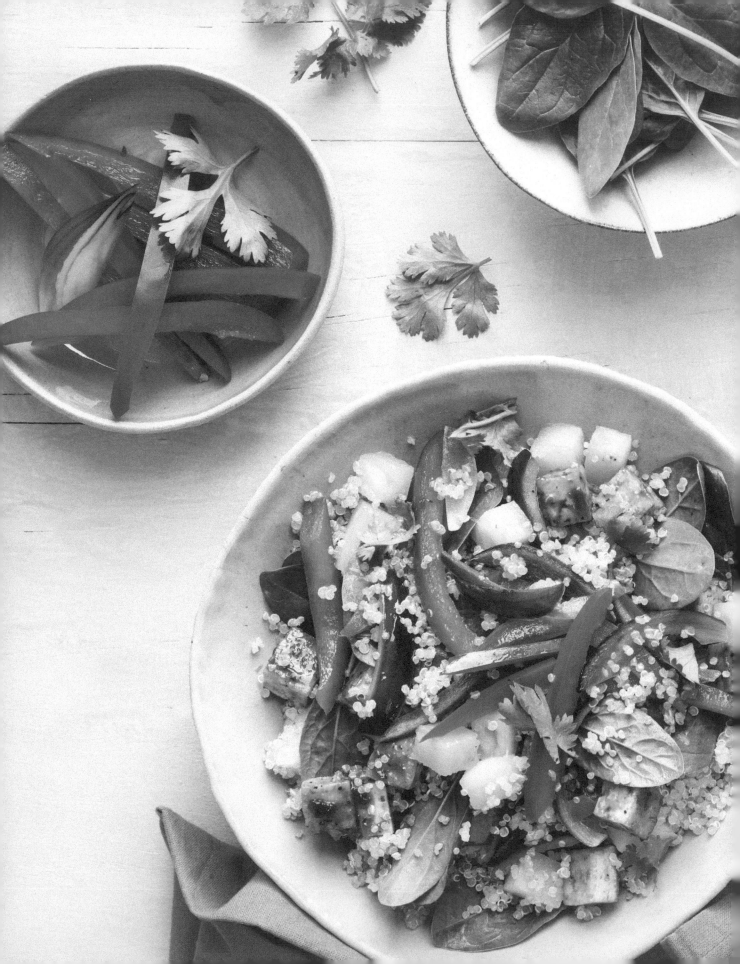

# THE
# Simply
# Vegan
## COOKBOOK

### Easy, Healthy, Fun, and Filling
### Plant-Based Recipes *Anyone* Can Cook

**DUSTIN HARDER**

Creator and Host of *The Vegan Roadie*

Foreword by Melissa d'Arabian,
author and *Food Network* host

Photography by Nadine Greeff

ROCKRIDGE
PRESS

Photography by Nadine Greeff
Author photo © Samantha Whetstone
Design by Christy Sheppard Knell

ISBN: Print 978-1-62315-926-9 | eBook 978-1-62315-927-6

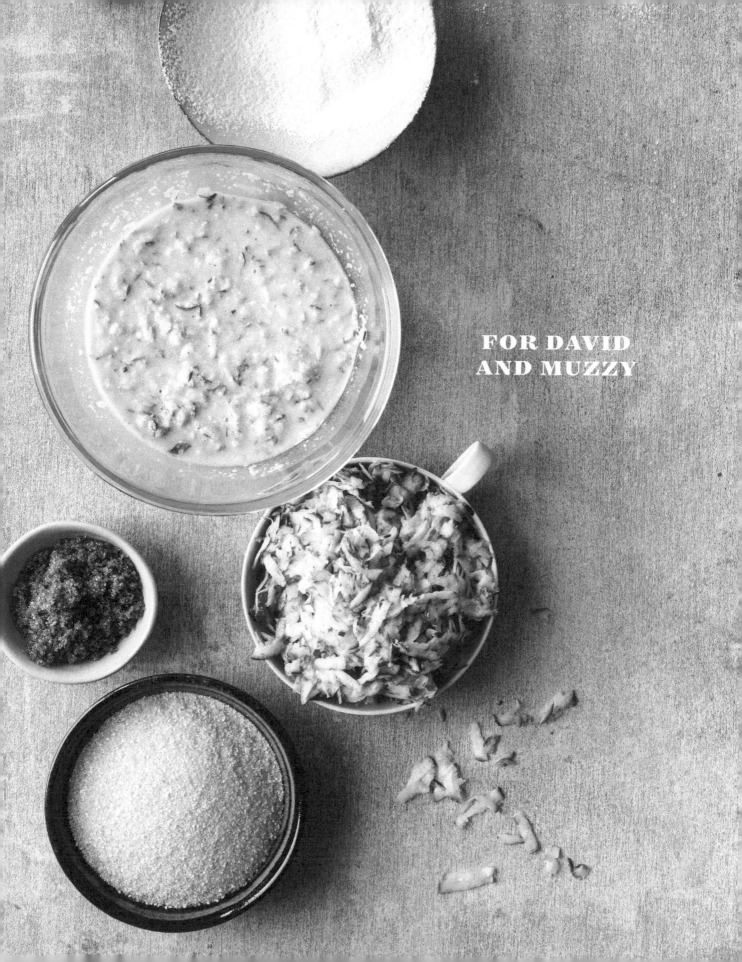

FOR DAVID
AND MUZZY

# Contents

# CHAPTER 3. BEANS

# CHAPTER 4. LENTILS

# CHAPTER 5. GRAINS

# CHAPTER 6. BROCCOLI & CAULIFLOWER

## CHAPTER 7. ROOT VEGETABLES

## CHAPTER 8. TOFU

## CHAPTER 9. SQUASH

# CHAPTER 10. AVOCADO

# CHAPTER 11. MUSHROOMS

# CHAPTER 12. SIMPLE SWEETS

## CHAPTER 13. KITCHEN STAPLES

# Foreword

A dog introduced me to Dustin, it's true. You might think a cooking show or an evening of fine dining would have brought us together, but it was a Broadway performance of *Annie*. After the show, I went backstage with my family to meet the rescue dog that played the role of Sandy, and I also met Dustin. We immediately connected over our love of animals, people, and food (of course). It was as if we'd been longtime pals reunited after years apart. Since that day, I've loved watching Dustin's influence in the food world grow.

Full disclosure: I'm not vegan. However, I certainly do rely on a diet filled with whole, plant-based foods. I'm a busy working mom, so most of my meals need to be easy, affordable, and nutritious. These recipes taste amazing and are so, so easy to make. If Dustin weren't there to remind me that the food is vegan, I'm not sure it'd even occur to me. When he told me he was writing a book that would make his vegan fans feel right at home while also welcoming in the slew of folks who want to eat more plant-based diets, I knew he'd nail it.

*If you are a seasoned vegan,* you'll love Dustin's creative take on well-loved favorites (try his Cauliflower Alfredo Your Way, page 111) as well as recipes that might surprise you, such as Avocado Breakfast Pizza (page 179) and Salted Coconut–Almond Fudge (page 214). Nothing is overly fussy. Dustin's experience cooking on the road has translated into an ability to create dishes that don't involve a lot of, well, dishes. Busy folks, rejoice! These recipes are accessible; doable, but never boring.

*If you are new to veganism*, or if you're simply looking to increase your intake of vegetables, Dustin is your perfect guide. Try his Simple Spinach and Artichoke Flatbread (page 23) or Kentucky Baked Cauliflower (page 113). As if the recipes weren't enough, Dustin gives helpful background on essential ingredients, equipping readers with a useful working knowledge of them. Here Dustin's recipes share much more than just a single dish. Readers get context and walk away from this cookbook with the confidence to play around in the kitchen and come out victorious. Dustin gives home cooks the courage—and encouragement—to step away from the recipes and try their hand at putting together a balanced, plant-based plate on any given weeknight.

Food is never just about fueling our bodies with calories and nutrients. It's about feeding our souls and connecting ourselves with each other and the world around us. In other words, it matters that Dustin's recipes aren't just foolproof, creative, and tasty, but that they are written with love and the desire to share his favorite meals with us. Making his recipes has me simultaneously missing Dustin's presence around my table and feeling like a little bit of him is sitting in our dining room, squarely among my daughters, who all adore him and would beg to sit next to him. Happily, this book brings Dustin to all of our tables, including yours.

MELISSA D'ARABIAN
*Food Network* host, columnist, and author of *Ten Dollar Dinners: 140 Recipes & Tips to Elevate Simple, Fresh Meals Any Night of the Week* and *Supermarket Healthy: Recipes and Know-How for Eating Well Without Spending a Lot*

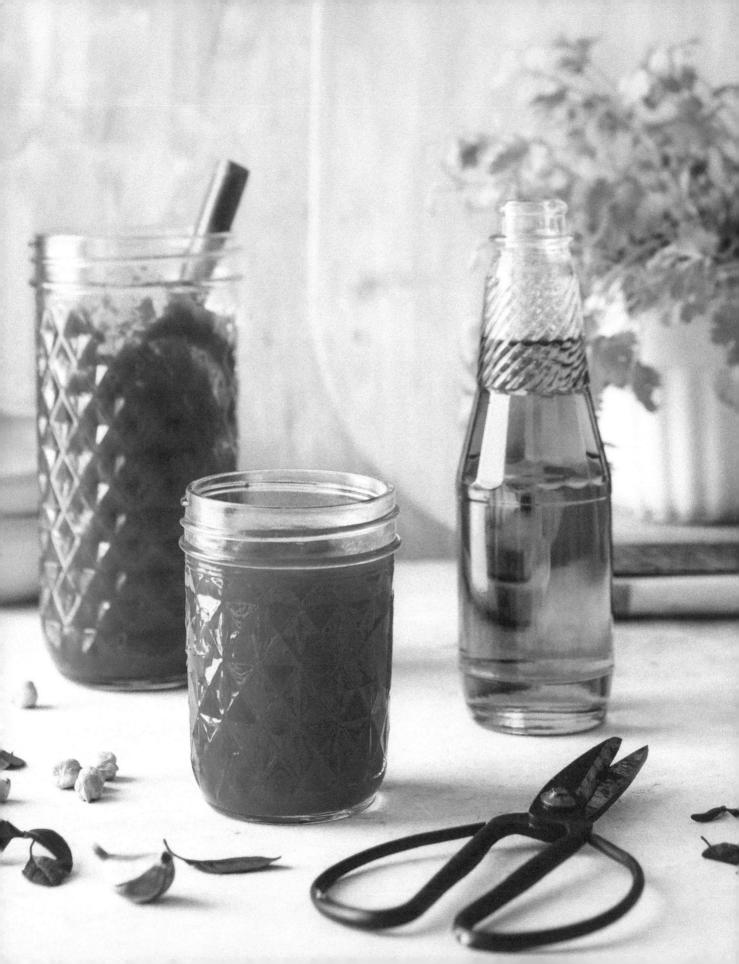

# CHAPTER 1

# Vegan Made Easy

*Fun* and *joy*—these are two words I hope you will keep in mind as you start to explore the world of vegan cooking. Food is not meant to be intimidating; on the contrary, it's meant to nourish our bodies and enlighten our senses. That doesn't sound so scary to me.

With this book, you'll probably be trying foods you've never considered before and perhaps cooking things in a different style than you have in the past. You might also find that you've been cooking things all along that you didn't realize were vegan. Surprise! The joys of veganism include discovering that Oreo cookies are vegan, and that you don't need to buy a $400 blender to become a kitchen warrior in your own home.

When you start investigating vegan options, remember that this is *your* journey, not anyone else's! I applaud your curiosity by simply opening this book. Be mindful that in finding recipes and plant-based products you love, loving everything is not a given. That's the way the eggless cookie crumbles—vegan or not. But that doesn't mean meatless Monday isn't for you. It just means *that* meatless Monday wasn't for you. Dust yourself off, flip this book open, and let your finger land on whichever recipe the page falls open to. That's your recipe for tonight. That's *simply vegan*.

## WHY THIS BOOK?

My sister has been saying for years, "I wish I could go vegan but it all seems so hard. I don't know what all these ingredients are. If only I had you to cook for me every day." I wrote this book for her and the millions of people like her—and most importantly, the person I was 10 years ago, when I decided to give eating vegan a go.

It was hard then for me, too. I was intimidated and overwhelmed by new ingredients. What did they taste like? Where could I buy them? It made me want to hang it all up and pour cow's milk on my cereal again. It seemed there was no other approach than "all or nothing." But then I relaxed, took a deep breath, and started small, with foods I knew. Suddenly, what started as a challenge turned into a party. I was having a blast in the kitchen recreating dishes I was most familiar with, with just a few adjustments. I want you to have that experience, too.

In my original video series, *The Vegan Roadie*, I have made it a priority to show on camera the one thing that everybody wants: delicious food. This book is no different. As a chef, I have taken the techniques I learned in culinary school, restaurant recipe development, and working with chefs across the miles while filming my show, and simplified them to create easy at-home versions of foods you will recognize and you already adore. These pages are jammed with 150 recipes that anyone can enjoy. They are simple, delicious, and just so happen to be vegan.

Each recipe in this book was created with compassion and joy. I hope you will find balance with ingredients handpicked for your enjoyment throughout these pages. Allow yourself to play with your food. I firmly believe that cooking should come from a place of love and curiosity.

# WHY THESE FOODS?

The recipe chapters are organized around main ingredients. These are ingredients that most commonly pop up in vegan recipes and work well in a variety of cooking methods. I organized things this way so that if you are at the supermarket or venture to the farmers' market and happen upon a vegetable or grain you want to try, you have a quick way to find plenty of recipes for it. I also did it in case you have a favorite ingredient but want some new ideas. Say you love spinach; there is a chapter on greens with five recipes just for spinach, including two variations on each recipe. That means 15 spinach recipes to expand your culinary repertoire. The same goes for many other common greens in that chapter.

Most importantly, the ingredients that are central to the chapters in this book form the building blocks of a solid vegan diet. It's a rewarding experience to build your own meal with enticing ingredients that create a fully realized nutritional profile. I want you to have fun with your food, but I also want you to feel amazing after you eat it. That's one of the perks of eating plants.

Most of these foods, aside from some grains and a few perishable items, should be found along the perimeter of your local supermarket. Have you ever taken a close look at the layout of your neighborhood superstore? All the fresh vegetables and fruits are on the perimeter. If you usually spend the majority of your time shopping in the middle of the supermarket and you want to change that, this book is for you.

Years of personal research and hands-on experience traveling 110,000 miles back and forth across the United States (that equals 14 cross-country trips, by the way), and visiting every type of grocery store from Manhattan to Kansas City, Albuquerque to Seattle, have shown me what is most accessible to the greatest number of people. No matter where you are on your food journey, this book offers foods that won't require you to place an order online or drive to that one health food store the next town over. You can shop close to home and still provide healthful, balanced meals for yourself, your family, and your friends. A few recipes call for miso paste, tahini, or nutritional yeast—but only a handful, I promise! If you are truly a novice to vegan cooking, I encourage you to get excited about these ingredients, because they will certainly come in handy as you expand your cooking catalogue. Or you could just skip those recipes, for now, and start with what is familiar.

## A Note About Nuts

Nuts—oh man, do I love nuts! As far as I'm concerned, cashews are the universe's gift to the plant-based culinary world. From nut butters to dreamy cheese sauces, nuts are the foundation for many vegan recipes. There are some brilliant books dedicated to nuts in vegan cuisine, and I highly recommend you invest in a nut book or two if you decide to delve deeper. There won't be a separate chapter for nuts; you will find them throughout this book as a primary ingredient for easy sauces, dressings, and toppings. They're also in some of the staples in chapter 13. But don't worry, I'll do my best to include nut-free variations whenever possible for those with allergies!

## WHAT TO EXPECT

I kept the equipment and tools used in these recipes to a bare minimum; standard pots, pans, and baking sheets do the trick for almost everything. While vegan cookbooks often rely on high-speed blenders and food processors, these recipes were tested on the kind of standard blender that is sold in mainstream department stores. Any blender you have will get the job done.

For every main recipe in this book, I give you two variations, so you can take favorites and mix them up, add a little pizzazz to leftovers for lunch the next day, or even mix and match to add your own creative flair.

I'm a visual fella, so the recipes in this book have these little icons to guide you:

**GF** Gluten-free
**NF** Nut-free
**SF** Soy-free
**30** 30 minutes or fewer

# Neat Cheats

We're fortunate that vegan staples are becoming more widely available in stores, and that's what I refer to here as "neat cheats." I love my meat alternatives and bottled vegan ranch dressing just as much as I love making my own staples. I have developed recipes for restaurants where every staple is store-bought, and others where the staff is literally squeezing almond milk out of a nut bag at 4 a.m. I can appreciate it all, but let's be real: If you picked up a cookbook with the word *simply* in the title, I'm guessing you don't have the patience or desire to whip up a batch of homemade mayonnaise every time you want to use some on a sandwich. And that is okay.

If you do buy instead of make, be sure to read the ingredients labels. In general, I avoid items with ingredients I can't pronounce or items with lengthy lists of ingredients. While chapter 13 includes recipes for pantry staples that I think are worth making yourself, you should feel free to purchase your favorite store-bought alternatives instead. Keep things as simple as you want them to be. You're the chef.

What follows are, in my opinion, vegan foods you can feel good about buying. See page 235 for specific brand recommendations:

## CHEESE

Vegan cheese has advanced by leaps and bounds in the past few years, and it's exciting to see companies keep improving on their original recipes. Look and you shall find vegan cheese shreds, cheese blocks, cheese slices, you name it. There are different versions based on soy, tofu, cashews, and so on. Some have a sharper or a milder flavor, just like cheese made from cow's milk. And similarly, it's trial and error to find brands that you like best. Ready-made cheese sauce can be a bit harder to find, so I've included my favorite cheese sauce recipe on page 224. As for grated Parmesan cheese, there are many good brands, but the challenge is availability. If you can't find it, it couldn't be simpler to make—see page 230.

## HUMMUS

While homemade hummus is unbelievably easy to make, there are plenty of great store-bought options for everything from plain hummus to black bean hummus to edamame hummus. Who ever said the chickpea had to be the king of hummus?

## MAYONNAISE

Mayo has taken off when it comes to companies battling it out for the best vegan version. There are many good options to choose from, and the ingredients lists are blessedly short. Vegan mayo is generally labeled "vegan," making it easy to spot.

## MEAT ALTERNATIVES

The cheat of all cheats. Sure, you can make a delicious burger patty from scratch with ease, and I will show you how on page 56. But if you are having a cookout and you forgot that your daughter's best friend is now vegan and you want to be the host with the most, options are plentiful these days. Try to keep it non-GMO. For those with a gluten sensitivity, meat alternatives can be tricky, but not impossible. May the fierce be with you.

## SALAD DRESSING

Companies have been diligently making progress to offer consumers flavors we know and love, like blue cheese and ranch. Not for nothing, but don't forget to look at the labels of dressings you already buy. You never know . . . maybe it's vegan and you didn't even notice!

## SOUR CREAM

I offer a quick recipe on page 222, but there are times when you just want to throw together a last-minute taco night without messing up the blender. One less thing to clean, right?

## YOGURT

There are several vegan brands on the market these days that are dangerously delicious. As with vegan cheeses, they are based on a range of ingredients—soy, coconut, cashews, and more—to suit your tastes and dietary needs. Store-bought yogurt can be heavy on the sugar, so if that's important to you, be mindful when tossing your new favorite vegan yogurt into your shopping cart!

Think of the recipes here as stepping stones. Once you have mastered them, I encourage you to move on to other books that do incorporate ingredients that might be unfamiliar to you. But for now, start simple, get excited, feed your hunger, keep an open mind, and—above all else—have fun!

## THE COMPLETE VEGAN PLATE

To reap the benefits of a healthy diet—such as normal blood pressure, lots of energy, and a reduced risk of developing heart disease, diabetes, and certain types of cancer—it's important to eat a wide variety of fruits, veggies, beans, whole grains, and other wholesome plant-based foods. Big surprise, huh? The good news here is that the phrase "easier said than done" does not apply; doing this on a vegan diet is just as easily done as it is said. A complete vegan plate consists of a good variety of foods, like grains, beans, legumes, and vegetables. It is considered complete because all these different foods together provide the various vitamins, minerals, and nutrients we need to fuel our bodies.

The thing most people new to the vegan diet worry about is a word that everyone loves to toss around like jokes at a comedy roast: *protein*. But unless you are doing some serious sports training and need to up your protein intake, it's nearly impossible *not* to get enough. I have done fitness-training programs where I did indeed require an increase in protein and, as a vegan, I figured it out. But if you're not actively training for an endurance or strength-training event, you probably don't need to concern yourself with "getting enough" protein. Almost every food contains protein, so the important thing is to eat a variety of foods every day.

That being said, what is a complete vegan plate? You'll see a recipe in chapter 2 that I call GGB Bowl (page 28). That stands for grains, greens, and beans. When you combine grains, greens, and beans, you get a variety of nutrients and—wait for it—a complete protein. You can then add more veggies, grains, or even protein, as you like. It can be that easy.

At the beginning of the grains (chapter 5), greens (chapter 2), and beans (chapter 3) chapters I give a quick how-to for making a basic batch of each, and some of the recipes in the chapters use those basic batches to create full meals. Once you get comfortable cooking these basics, you can also change up your technique to suit your health needs; for instance, when it says to sauté in oil you can sauté in water or vegetable broth for lower fat content. There are lots of ways to trim numbers and maintain nutrients, but that's a different book. This one gives you the quick and easy methods you need for a surefire delicious finish.

The bottom line here is to pay attention to what you need; everyone's body is different. Find what your balance is. When I'm paying attention to numbers I find great use in smartphone apps like Lose It! and MyFitnessPal. In this day and age we have all the tools we need to take the stress out of eating, making meals that are great for our everyday health and wellness goals simple and satisfying.

## MAKE IT FUN

It's easy to overthink cooking and eating in a new way. But really, all you need is the desire to incorporate some meatless meals into your life. Try not to overthink it, and go one meal at a time. How often you eat vegan is completely up to you, but I do hope this book becomes a resource for you. I mentioned fun and joy in the intro. Keep that in mind whenever you decide to tie those apron strings—or slip on your high heels, or dance around singing into a spatula in your underwear while you cook. I'm not here to judge. But please, if you are in your undies, be careful around the stove! Fun is the goal whenever I step into the kitchen, and it's why I wrote this book. I firmly believe cooking can be fun and easy, which makes it undeniably enjoyable.

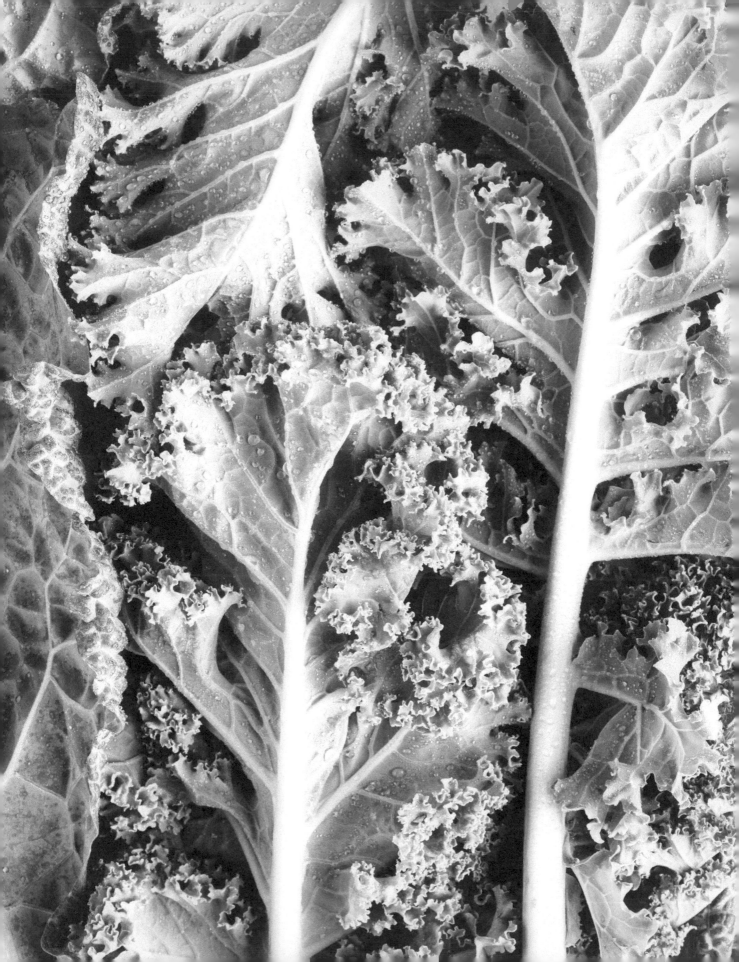

# CHAPTER 2
# Greens

I think we all know that greens are beneficial for us. Just the same, I'm certain we can also agree that most of us struggle to get the big G into our diets. This chapter is full of easy, delicious options for you to mix and match and make complete plates that include greens.

This chapter only scratches the surface on leafy greens, offering ways to incorporate them with ease into your diet. Like any food, the more you cook your greens, the less nutrients they retain. That's why you will find both raw salads and warm dishes in this chapter. Whenever you can, add a serving of raw greens to a meal to make it more nutrient-dense. This is where smoothies come in handy for me.

If you don't like your greens raw, including cooked greens in your diet is still certainly more nutritious than many other choices you can make in terms of what's on your plate. Until you get comfortable enough to experiment on your own, use this chapter to stick with greens you are most likely familiar with—kale, spinach, cabbage, lettuce, and arugula. Then you can branch out into chard, collard greens, broccoli rabe, dandelion greens, and even the leafy tops of root vegetables, like beets and turnips and radishes—the parts you used to throw away. Not anymore! They're so tasty. Swap them in and out of the recipes here for different flavors and textures. So again, have fun (see the theme here?), play with your greens, pick up new ones you have never used before, and experiment.

# THE BASICS OF COOKING GREENS

Before we dive into specific recipes, I want to show you a couple of simple methods to prepare greens, and greens alone. You will find the fun of incorporating greens into recipes later in this chapter, but these methods will give you the confidence to cook greens on their own as well.

To start, thoroughly wash the greens and trim off the bottoms of the stems. For sturdier greens like chard and collards, you'll want to remove the stem completely. For slightly tougher greens like kale, you may have to detach the whole leaf from the center stem; you can use a knife or simply rip it off. For more delicate greens like baby spinach, there is no need to chop or remove stems.

### TO SAUTÉ

1 to 3 teaspoons olive oil

½ cup chopped onion (optional)

1 garlic clove, minced (optional)

1 bunch or 1 (5-ounce) package greens of your choice

½ teaspoon lemon juice or vinegar (optional)

**1.** Heat the oil in a large skillet over medium heat. Or, if you're cutting back on fat content, use water or vegetable broth, or a mixture of either with oil. Start with ¼ cup water or broth, and be mindful to keep adding liquid during the process to avoid burning.

**2.** Add the chopped onion, if using, and sauté for 3 minutes, or until soft.

**3.** If using garlic, add it now and sauté for 1 additional minute, or until fragrant.

**4.** Add the greens, in batches if space is limited, allowing the previous batch to cook down before adding more.

**5.** When all the greens have cooked and wilted, embellish with a dash of acid, such as lemon juice or your favorite vinegar, if desired.

### TO STEAM

Salt (optional)

1 bunch or 1 (5-ounce) package greens of your choice

**1.** Put a steamer basket in a large pot and add enough water so that it comes up to just beneath the steamer basket.

**2.** If desired, add some salt to the water. This will flavor the greens slightly.

**3.** Fill the steamer basket with greens, cover the pot, and bring the water to a boil over high heat.

**4.** Once the water is boiling, the greens will steam and wilt within 2 to 4 minutes.

**TIP:** *Use greens from either method in the GGB Bowl (page 28), serve cooked greens as a side dish with your favorite vegan protein, or throw them into a pasta dish of your own invention.*

# Blueberry Lemonade Smoothie

1 cup roughly chopped kale

¾ cup frozen blueberries

1 cup unsweetened soy or almond milk

Juice of 1 lemon

1 tablespoon maple syrup

SERVES 1 • PREP TIME: 5 MINUTES

My life drastically changed when I started sneaking greens into my morning smoothie. I could actually feel the difference in my body from getting nutrients that were broken down into the most digestible form. Honestly, I love smoothies so much, I suck them down like a milk-shake. With smoothies like these, I don't have to feel bad about that!

Combine all the ingredients in a blender and blend until smooth. Enjoy immediately.

**VARIATIONS**

**STRAWBERRY LEMONADE SMOOTHIE:** Replace the blueberries with 1 cup strawberries.

**TROPICAL SMOOTHIE:** Replace the blueberries with ½ cup mango chunks and ½ cup pineapple chunks.

**TIP:** *The amount of liquid depends on your blender and its speed, so you may need to use more milk. If you want to cut caloric content, use half milk and half water, or just water.*

# Mango Key Lime Pie Smoothie

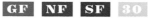

¼ avocado

1 cup baby spinach

½ cup frozen mango chunks

1 cup unsweetened soy or almond milk

Juice of 1 lime (preferably a Key lime, if you can find one!)

1 tablespoon maple syrup

SERVES 1 • PREP TIME: 5 MINUTES

We are gathered here today to witness the union of mangos and limes. If anyone has any objections, kindly keep your mouth shut. This drink is velvety smooth, with the perfect amount of tart and sweet, and who doesn't love pie for breakfast? This is pie you can feel good about.

Combine all the ingredients in a blender and blend until smooth. Enjoy immediately.

### VARIATIONS

**MANGO KEY LIME PIE SMOOTHIE BOWL:** Pour the smoothie into a cereal bowl. Top with granola, shredded coconut, and goji berries for a filling and healthful start to your morning.

**LEMON-LIME SMOOTHIE:** Replace the mango with 1 frozen banana and use the juice of both 1 lemon and 1 lime.

**TIP:** *Use frozen fruit in smoothies to avoid having to add ice to make your smoothie thick and cold. Ice can water a smoothie down, resulting in a weaker flavor.*

# Almond Crunch Chopped Kale Salad

**GF** **30**

SERVES 4 • PREP TIME: 10 MINUTES • COOK TIME: 10 MINUTES

**FOR THE DRESSING**

¼ cup tahini

2 tablespoons Dijon mustard

2 tablespoons maple syrup

1 tablespoon lemon juice

¼ teaspoon salt

**FOR THE ALMOND CRUNCH**

½ cup finely chopped raw almonds

2 teaspoons soy sauce or
   gluten-free tamari

1 teaspoon maple syrup

¼ teaspoon sea salt

**FOR THE SALAD**

1 bunch lacinato kale, stemmed and
   roughly chopped

1 green apple, cored and thinly sliced

I love this salad because I can put it together quickly and it's loaded with flavor. I make the dressing first, so it is ready to go by the time my salad ingredients are prepared, and I can avoid the apple oxidizing and turning brown. This is one of my favorite dishes to take to a Fourth of July gathering; there are never any leftovers! My recipe calls for lacinato kale, also known as Tuscan or dinosaur kale. It's the one with the darker, narrower, flat leaves.

**1.** Preheat the oven to 325°F. Line a baking sheet with parchment paper.

**2.** *To make the dressing:* Whisk together all the dressing ingredients in a small bowl and set aside.

**3.** *To make the almond crunch:* Mix together all the almond crunch ingredients in a medium bowl and spread out evenly on the prepared baking sheet. Bake for 5 to 7 minutes, until slightly darker in color and crunchy. Let cool for 3 minutes.

**4.** *To make the salad:* In a large bowl, mix together the kale and apples. Toss with the dressing and top with the almond crunch.

**VARIATIONS**

**TOFU-KALE TAHINI WRAP:** Add some Basic Baked Tofu (page 137), throw it into a wrap with this salad, and you have a complete lunch! The wrap holds up nicely even with the dressing, because the lacinato kale is so sturdy.

**SALTED CHOPPED KALE TOAST:** Avocado toast is popular, but pile this on top of your toast and sprinkle with some flaked sea salt to wow your brunch guests.

**TIP:** *If you want to slice the apples in advance, toss them in the juice of ½ lemon to keep them from browning.*

# Darn Good Caesar Salad

## FOR THE DRESSING

½ cup walnuts

½ cup water

3 tablespoons olive oil

Juice of ½ lime

1 tablespoon white miso paste

1 teaspoon soy sauce or gluten-free tamari

1 teaspoon Dijon mustard

1 teaspoon garlic powder

¼ teaspoon sea salt

½ teaspoon black pepper

## FOR THE SALAD

2 heads romaine lettuce, chopped

1 cup cherry tomatoes, halved

Walnut Parmesan (page 230) or store-bought vegan Parmesan, for garnish

Vegan croutons, for garnish (optional)

SERVES 4 TO 6 • PREP TIME: 10 MINUTES

I was always miffed at the lack of Caesar salad options at vegan restaurants, although thankfully, that has started to change. After I created this dressing, I served this salad to anyone who came over. It is the perfect starter for a dinner party with a variety of palates to please.

**1.** *To make the dressing:* In a blender, combine all the dressing ingredients and blend until almost smooth, about 2 minutes. It's okay if this dressing is slightly chunky, which is more like a classic Caesar dressing texture.

**2.** *To make the salad:* In a large bowl, toss the lettuce with half of the dressing. Add more as desired. Divide among serving plates and top with the tomatoes and Parmesan. Finish the salad off with croutons, if desired.

## VARIATIONS

**CHICKEN CAESAR SALAD:** Add vegan grilled chicken strips to recreate the classic.

**CHICKEN CAESAR WRAP:** Divide the salad mixture among 4 to 6 large (10-inch) burrito tortillas. Wrap it up with vegan chicken strips for a very satisfying lunch on the go.

**TIP:** *Easily make your own croutons by cutting up vegan bread into cubes, tossing with melted vegan butter or olive oil, and seasoning with salt and pepper. Spread out on a parchment-lined baking sheet and bake at 350°F for 6 to 8 minutes, until browned, tossing once halfway through. Add some Italian seasoning with the salt and pepper for a little extra flavor. If you struggle to find miso paste for this recipe, it's okay to omit it and use in its place 1 tablespoon of Dijon mustard (this is in addition to the Dijon already called for). But if you can find miso, use it for the tastiest outcome!*

# Sunshine Fiesta Salad

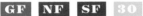   

**GF** **NF** **SF** 30

**SERVES 4 · PREP TIME: 15 MINUTES**

**FOR THE VINAIGRETTE**

Juice of 2 limes

1 tablespoon olive oil

1 tablespoon maple syrup or agave

¼ teaspoon sea salt

**FOR THE SALAD**

2 cups cooked quinoa

1 tablespoon Taco Seasoning
(page 219) or store-bought taco
seasoning

2 heads romaine lettuce,
roughly chopped

1 (15-ounce) can black beans, rinsed
and drained

1 cup cherry tomatoes, halved

1 cup frozen (and thawed) or fresh
corn kernels

1 avocado, peeled, pitted, and diced

4 scallions, thinly sliced

12 tortilla chips, crushed

This salad is full of fresh ingredients that are brought together by a super-simple lime vinaigrette. There are a couple of steps that take this from dull to delicious—and they're totally worth it. Using the variations, you can make this salad as deluxe or basic as you wish. I say go for the deluxe! It's my sister's favorite salad and therefore named after her—yes, my sister's name is Sunshine. Shockingly, my parents were not hippies.

**1.** *To make the vinaigrette:* In a small bowl, whisk together all the vinaigrette ingredients.

**2.** *To make the salad:* In a medium bowl, mix together the quinoa and taco seasoning.

**3.** In a large bowl, toss the romaine with the vinaigrette. Divide among 4 bowls.

**4.** Top each bowl with equal amounts quinoa, beans, tomatoes, corn, avocado, scallions, and crushed tortillas chips.

### VARIATIONS

**TACO SALAD DELUXE:** Omit the quinoa. Top the salad with vegan beef crumbles, sour cream, Guacamole (page 172), pepitas (roasted pumpkin seeds), and vegan cheddar shreds.

**TACO NIGHT:** To make any night a taco night, make the Taco Salad Deluxe above. Purchase some soft or hard taco shells, or both, and fill the shells with the taco salad ingredients. Heck, throw it all into a big taco shell bowl, if you can find one!

**TIP:** *I prefer to use frozen corn, but if you want to cut the corn straight off the cob, applause for you. If you are in the frozen category with me, I either thaw mine in the fridge overnight or set it in a bowl of hot water for a few minutes, then drain.*

# Cobb Salad with Portobello Bacon

 **GF** 30

2 heads romaine lettuce,
    finely chopped

1 pint cherry tomatoes, halved

1 avocado, peeled, pitted, and diced

1 cup frozen (and thawed) or fresh
    corn kernels

1 large cucumber, peeled and diced

Portobello Bacon (page 185) or
    store-bought vegan bacon

4 scallions, thinly sliced

Unhidden Valley Ranch Dressing
    (page 221) or store-bought vegan
    ranch dressing

SERVES 4 • PREP TIME: 15 MINUTES

This salad offers up a combination of fresh ingredients that complement one another and bring out the best of what's in the garden. Top with some decadent ranch and the added crisp of bacon for a light lunch that won't leave you hungry.

**1.** Scatter a layer of romaine in the bottom of each of 4 salad bowls. With the following ingredients, create lines that cross the top of the romaine, in this order: tomatoes, avocado, corn, cucumber, and portobello bacon.

**2.** Sprinkle with the scallions and drizzle with ranch dressing.

### VARIATIONS

**CHICKEN COBB SALAD:** Use your favorite vegan chicken, cut into ½-inch cubes, as an additional line on top of the lettuce.

**PROTEIN COBB SALAD:** Punch up the protein by adding some beans, hemp seeds, or chia seeds—or all three!

**TIP:** *I like to keep a batch of Portobello Bacon on hand to put on salads, sandwiches, and pizzas. Most of the time it doesn't make it into any recipe, though, as I find myself munching on it as a snack.*

# Apple, Pecan, and Arugula Salad

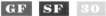 **GF** **SF** 30

Juice of 1 lemon

2 tablespoons olive oil

1 tablespoon maple syrup

2 pinches sea salt

1 (5-ounce) package arugula

1 cup frozen (and thawed) or fresh corn kernels

½ red onion, thinly sliced

2 apples (preferably Gala or Fuji), cored and sliced

½ cup chopped pecans

¼ cup dried cranberries

**SERVES 4 • PREP TIME: 10 MINUTES**

I used to dislike arugula, until one day it came on the side with a sandwich I ordered. It was dressed simply in olive oil with tomatoes . . . and to my surprise, I loved it! I want to offer you this possibility for the joy I found in arugula, with a simple salad that I feel has elements that complement one another.

**1.** In a small bowl, whisk together the lemon juice, oil, maple syrup, and salt.

**2.** In a large bowl, combine the arugula, corn, red onion, and apples. Add the lemon-juice mixture and toss to combine.

**3.** Divide evenly among 4 plates and top with the pecans and cranberries.

## VARIATIONS

**APPLE, PECAN, AND ARUGULA SALAD WITH CHICKEN:** This light salad is nicely enhanced with the addition of grilled vegan chicken.

**FANTASTIC FANCY SANDWICH:** Serve this salad on a vegan baguette topped with hummus or mayo and Fast Feta (page 225).

**TIP:** *Apples turn brown once sliced. To avoid this, place them in either cold water or lemon juice until you are ready to use them. If you are making this salad and serving it right away, you don't have to worry about this.*

# Mexi Walnut and Sun-Dried Tomato Lettuce Wraps

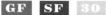

1 cup walnuts, roughly chopped

½ cup sun-dried tomatoes, roughly chopped (rinsed if packed in oil)

2 carrots, peeled and grated

1 celery stalk, thinly sliced

¼ cup roughly chopped fresh cilantro

2 teaspoons Taco Seasoning (page 219) or store-bought taco seasoning

Juice of ½ lime

2 teaspoons olive oil

2 teaspoons agave or maple syrup

Sea salt

6 to 12 Bibb lettuce leaves

2 scallions, thinly sliced

**SERVES 4 • PREP TIME: 15 MINUTES**

Said the walnut to the sun-dried tomato, "Lettuce get together." And so they shall. I love this mixture of sweet and tangy sun-dried tomatoes with the earthy and fruity flavor of the walnuts; with just a few spices and accompanying veggies, the combination can't be beat! This recipe comes together in a snap for an anytime meal or snack.

**1.** In a large bowl, toss together the walnuts, sun-dried tomatoes, carrots, celery, cilantro, taco seasoning, lime juice, oil, and agave. Mix well to combine. Season with salt, starting with just a couple pinches and adding more if desired.

**2.** Scoop some of the mixture onto each lettuce leaf. Sprinkle with scallions and serve.

### VARIATIONS

**DESSERT LETTUCE WRAPS:** Omit the walnuts, sun-dried tomatoes, carrots, celery, cilantro, and taco seasoning (the first 6 ingredients). Instead, use 1 cup roughly chopped mango, 1 cup hulled and roughly chopped strawberries, and ¼ cup roughly chopped fresh basil. Mix with the lime juice, olive oil, and agave in a large bowl until well combined. Divide among the lettuce leaves and dust with organic confectioners' sugar.

**TOFU LETTUCE WRAPS:** Omit the walnuts and sun-dried tomatoes. Instead, use 1 (14-ounce block) extra-firm tofu, drained and crumbled. Mix with the remaining ingredients in a large bowl, divide among the lettuce leaves, and sprinkle with the scallions.

**TIP:** *Make all three variations for a party and leave the different fillings in bowls for guests to build their own wraps.*

# #kaledit Salt and Vinegar Kale Chips

   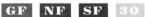

1 large bunch curly kale, stemmed and torn into 2- to 3-inch pieces (about 4 cups)

2 tablespoons apple cider vinegar

1 tablespoon olive oil

¾ teaspoon sea salt

**SERVES 2 • PREP TIME: 5 MINUTES • COOK TIME: 10 MINUTES**

Kale chips have come and gone; they were very popular and now seem to be forgotten. But I always keep this recipe in my back pocket. It's super simple and is still the life of the party when I put these chips out at gatherings. My kale chips bring all the boys to the yard!

1. Preheat the oven to 350°F. Line a large baking sheet or 2 small baking sheets with parchment paper.

2. Combine all the ingredients in a large bowl and massage everything together for 1 to 2 minutes, until the kale is soft and a darker green.

3. Spread the kale in a single layer on the prepared baking sheet(s). Do not pile the pieces on top of each other. Bake for 8 to 10 minutes, until the kale is crunchy.

4. Cool before serving. Store leftovers in a sealed container for up to 1 week.

## VARIATIONS

**DESSERT KALE CHIPS:** Omit the vinegar. Add 1 teaspoon vanilla extract, 1 teaspoon organic cane sugar, and ½ teaspoon ground cinnamon. Toss well to combine.

**CHEESE KALE CHIPS:** Omit the vinegar. Add 2 tablespoons Walnut Parmesan (page 230).

**TIP:** *After washing kale, dry it very thoroughly before dressing with the oil and vinegar (a salad spinner might help). Kale that is wet from water will not crisp up in the oven.*

# Simple Spinach and Artichoke Flatbread

SF 30

1½ cups raw cashews, soaked overnight or boiled for 10 minutes, and drained

1½ cups water

Juice of 1 lemon

2 garlic cloves, roughly chopped

1½ teaspoons onion powder

1½ teaspoons sea salt

1 (14-ounce) can quartered artichokes, rinsed, drained, and roughly chopped

1 (10-ounce) bag frozen spinach, thawed, drained, and squeezed dry

6 (6-inch) whole-wheat pita breads

6 teaspoons olive oil, divided

1 (8-ounce) package baby bella mushrooms, stemmed and sliced (optional)

Walnut Parmesan (page 230) or store-bought vegan Parmesan, for garnish

Red pepper flakes, for garnish

**SERVES 6 · PREP TIME: 10 MINUTES · COOK TIME: 15 MINUTES**

There is a pizza place in New York City called Artichoke Basille's that always has a long line out the door. I finally waited my turn one day and got a slice, and it was a slice of heaven. When I went vegan, I vowed to figure out a way to replicate that slice without all the cholesterol— or the use of a pizza oven. The original slice didn't have mushrooms, but I couldn't resist topping off this concoction of creamy goodness with some baby bellas!

**1.** Preheat the oven to 350°F. Line two baking sheets with parchment paper.

**2.** Combine the cashews, water, lemon juice, garlic, onion powder, and salt in a blender and blend until smooth. Pour the cashew mixture into a large mixing bowl. Add the artichokes. Now, double-check that your spinach is really and truly dry, because it will make your mixture watery if not. Then add the spinach and mix until well combined.

**3.** Brush each pita with 1 teaspoon of olive oil. Lay the pitas on the prepared baking sheets. Spread ½ cup of the spinach and artichoke mixture on each pita and top with the sliced baby bellas, if using.

**4.** Bake for 15 minutes, or until the edges start to turn golden brown. Top each flatbread with Parmesan and red pepper flakes. →

## VARIATIONS

**CLASSIC SPINACH-ARTICHOKE DIP:** Turn this into the life of the party! Bake the cashew and artichoke mixture in an oven-safe baking dish at 350°F for 25 minutes and top with Walnut Parmesan. Serve with crispy tortilla chips or warm bread.

**MINI PIZZAS:** Using burrito-size tortillas, cut out rounds with a 2½-inch biscuit cutter or round cookie cutter. Spray a muffin tin with nonstick cooking spray. Place a tortilla round in each muffin cup and top with a heaping tablespoon of the spinach-and-artichoke mixture. Bake at 350°F for 12 minutes. Remove from the oven and pop out each mini pizza with a fork. Sprinkle with Walnut Parmesan and red pepper flakes. Keep 'em coming, because your guests will devour these.

**TIP:** *If you don't have a brush to brush the oil over the pitas, drizzle the olive oil over the pitas and spread it with a clean paper towel.*

# Spinach, Tomato, and Orzo Soup

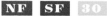  

1 tablespoon olive oil

1 onion, chopped

4 garlic cloves, minced

1 (14.5-ounce) can diced Italian tomatoes (preferably with oregano and basil)

4 cups low-sodium vegetable broth

4 cups water

1 teaspoon sea salt

1 teaspoon black pepper

1 pound uncooked orzo pasta

1 (5-ounce) package baby spinach

SERVES 6 TO 8 • PREP TIME: 10 MINUTES • COOK TIME: 20 MINUTES

I could dedicate an entire cookbook to soup. It's not something I typically order when I go out to eat, but I love to make it at home on a Sunday night from things I have hanging out in my refrigerator or pantry from the week before. Soup is a great way to use up produce before it goes bad, and it sets you up to have some quick meals ready for the week ahead.

**1.** Heat the oil in a large stockpot over medium heat. Add the onion and sauté for 3 minutes, or until soft. Add the garlic and sauté for 1 additional minute, or until fragrant. Add the tomatoes with their juice, broth, water, salt, and pepper. Cover the pot and bring to a boil. Reduce the heat to a simmer.

**2.** Add the orzo and cook, uncovered, for 9 minutes, or until the pasta is tender. Turn off the heat and stir in the spinach until wilted.

## VARIATIONS

**CHICKEN, SPINACH, AND ORZO SOUP:** Add diced vegan chicken when adding the pasta to the pot.

**SPINACH AND TOMATO STEW:** Sauté 1 cup chopped carrots and ½ cup chopped celery with the onion. Add 2 russet potatoes (peeled and cut into ½-inch cubes) when adding the broth and water. Cook for 15 to 18 minutes, until the potatoes are fork-tender. Reduce the orzo to ½ pound, and add it for the last 9 minutes of cooking.

**TIP:** *Your orzo will continue to cook in the hot liquid, so don't overcook it by letting the water continue to simmer. When the pasta sits for a few minutes after it's removed from the heat, it reaches its perfect texture and doubles in size.*

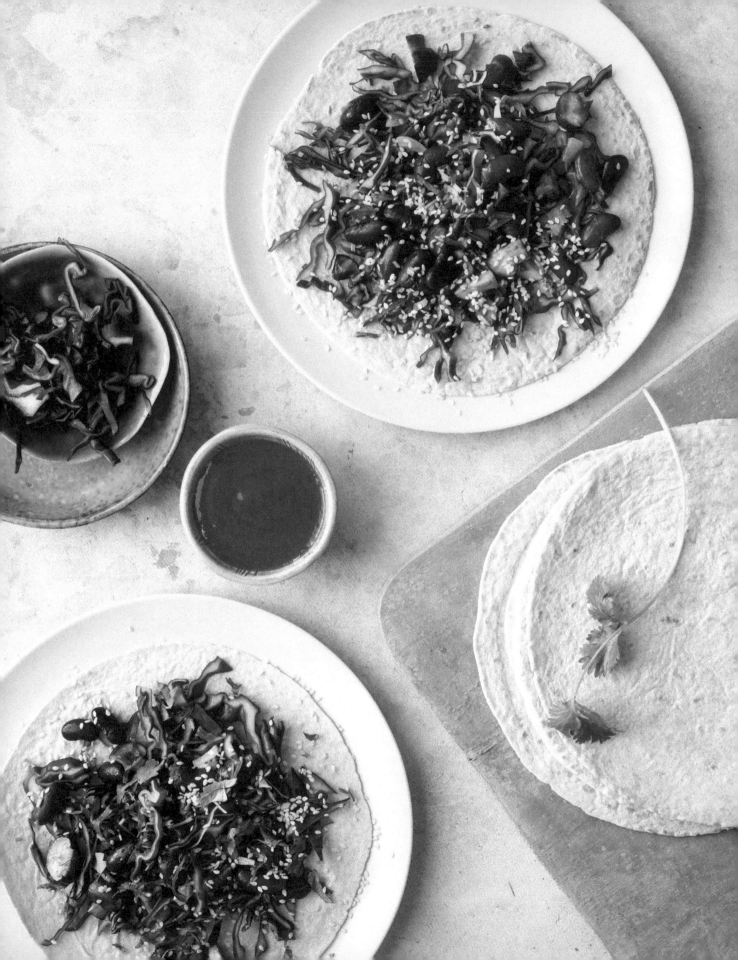

# Sheet-Pan Tacos with Cilantro and Cabbage Slaw

**GF** **NF**

SERVES 8 • PREP TIME: 10 MINUTES • COOK TIME: 25 MINUTES

**FOR THE SLAW**

3 cups thinly sliced purple cabbage

¼ cup Mayonnaise (page 223) or store-bought vegan mayonnaise

Juice of ½ lemon

¼ cup chopped fresh cilantro

½ teaspoon sea salt

**FOR THE TACOS**

1 (15-ounce) can pink or red beans, rinsed and drained

1 (8-ounce) package baby bella or white button mushrooms, stemmed and diced

1 onion, thinly sliced

1 tablespoon olive oil

½ teaspoon sea salt

½ teaspoon black pepper

8 (6-inch) corn tortillas

Sriracha sauce

1 tablespoon white sesame seeds, for garnish (optional)

I would like to quickly say that we are sending a terrible message to our children with "Taco Tuesdays." I trust you to do the right thing, and you can start now with this recipe. Let every child know that tacos are an acceptable form of awesome on any day of the week.

**1.** Preheat the oven to 400°F. Line a baking sheet with parchment paper.

**2.** *To make the slaw:* In a large bowl, toss the cabbage with the mayonnaise, lemon juice, cilantro, and salt.

**3.** *To make the tacos:* In another large bowl, combine the beans, mushrooms, onion, oil, salt, and pepper. Mix well and spread out on the prepared baking sheet. Bake for 10 minutes, toss with a spatula, and bake for an additional 10 minutes.

**4.** Lay the tortillas directly on top of the mushroom mixture and bake for 2 more minutes to warm them. Using tongs, transfer the tortillas to a plate.

**5.** On each tortilla, spread a layer of the mushroom mixture, followed by the slaw, and then a drizzle of sriracha. Sprinkle with sesame seeds, if desired.

**VARIATIONS**

**TROPICAL TACOS:** Replace 1 cup of the cabbage with 1 cup roughly chopped mango or pineapple.

**CILANTRO AND CABBAGE SLAW BOWL:** Instead of using corn tortillas, divide the slaw-and-mushroom mixture among 4 bowls, add ½ cup cooked rice or quinoa and 1 cup chopped romaine lettuce to each bowl, and sprinkle with hemp and chia seeds for an extra dose of protein.

**TIP:** *To serve these tacos upright at a party, set the filled tacos side by side in a 1-quart baking dish. They should fit snugly and be easily accessible for guests to enjoy.*

# GGB Bowl

 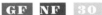 

**GF  NF  30**

2 teaspoons olive oil

1 cup cooked brown rice, quinoa, or your grain of choice

1 (15-ounce) can chickpeas or your beans of choice, rinsed and drained

1 bunch spinach or kale, stemmed and roughly chopped

1 tablespoon soy sauce or gluten-free tamari

Sea salt

Black pepper

**SERVES 2 · PREP TIME: 10 MINUTES · COOK TIME: 5 MINUTES**

Here it is, my beloved grains, greens, and beans bowl. Feel free to tweak it as you will; this recipe is open to interpretation and personal preference. Use it to expand your ingredient knowledge, knowing that you can count on a complete protein at the end each time!

**1.** In a large skillet, heat the oil over medium heat. Add the rice, beans, and greens and stir continuously until the greens have wilted and everything is heated through, 3 to 5 minutes.

**2.** Drizzle in the soy sauce, mix to combine, and season with salt and pepper.

## VARIATIONS

**ROASTED VEGETABLE BOWL:** Add roasted vegetables to your GGB bowl. Use 1 cup sliced carrots and 1 zucchini, halved and sliced, for some color. Toss with 1 tablespoon olive oil and salt and pepper to taste, and roast at 400°F for 20 minutes, tossing the vegetables halfway through.

**PROTEIN POWER GGB BOWL:** Add a vegan protein like tofu, tempeh, or other meat alternative to the bowl. Sprinkle with hemp and/or chia seeds for a protein-packed meal.

**TIP:** *Be adventurous and mix and match to your liking. Make it as is at first, and then let your creative side explore and expand. Find a new green you want to try? Use that. A bean you have always been curious about? Use that. Always wanted to make that pot of couscous? Now is the time! It's your kitchen and your bowl, so take charge and make food that piques your palate.*

# Red, White, and Green Pasta Bowl

 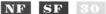 

1 tablespoon olive oil

1 onion, chopped

½ cup roughly chopped
    sun-dried tomatoes

1 (8-ounce) package baby bella
    or white button mushrooms,
    stemmed and sliced

6 garlic cloves, minced

¼ teaspoon sea salt

¼ teaspoon black pepper

¼ teaspoon red pepper flakes

½ cup low-sodium vegetable broth

1 bunch kale, stemmed and
    roughly chopped

3 cups farfalle, cooked

1 (15-ounce) can cannellini beans,
    rinsed and drained

Walnut Parmesan (page 230) or
    store-bought vegan Parmesan,
    for garnish (optional)

Chopped fresh parsley,
    for garnish (optional)

**SERVES 6 • PREP TIME: 10 MINUTES • COOK TIME: 15 MINUTES**

I have such a love-hate relationship with pasta. Carbs tend to do that to us, eh? When I was a kid, one of my favorite meals was a big bowl of spaghetti loaded with butter and processed Parmesan cheese. Thankfully, I've grown to love my vegetables as an adult, but even better, I find joy mixing them into my pasta. So I'm eliminating the hate and making it a big old bowl of love! I hope you can do the same with this recipe, where veggies, beans, and kale join pasta bow ties.

**1.** Heat the oil in a large skillet over medium heat. Add the onion, sun-dried tomatoes, and mushrooms and sauté until the onion is soft and the mushrooms have reduced in size, about 5 minutes. Add the garlic, salt, black pepper, and red pepper flakes and cook for 1 additional minute, or until fragrant.

**2.** Slowly add the broth to the pan and stir in the kale. Cover and simmer for 5 minutes, or until the kale is completely wilted.

**3.** Stir in the cooked pasta and beans and cook for 2 minutes, or until heated through.

**4.** Serve in shallow bowls and garnish with Parmesan and chopped fresh parsley, if desired.

### VARIATIONS

**SAUSAGE FARFALLE BOWL:** Omit the mushrooms. Add 3 links of your favorite vegan Italian sausage, sliced, for a heartier dish or to satiate your carnivorous friends.

**MARINARA AND FARFALLE:** This dish is intended to be a drier pasta. Add your favorite store-bought sauce or Magnificent Marinara (page 231) if you prefer more gravy with your pasta.

**TIP:** *Sun-dried tomatoes that are packed in oil are fine for this—just take out the amount of tomatoes you need and rinse them off. For a flavor boost, use 1 tablespoon of the oil from the jar of tomatoes instead of the olive oil called for in the recipe.*

# The Cabbage Patch Bowl

2 medium russet potatoes, cut into
½-inch cubes

2 tablespoons olive oil, divided

½ teaspoon sea salt, divided

½ teaspoon black pepper, divided

2 cups bite-size broccoli florets

4 cups shredded purple cabbage

1 tablespoon tamari

2 cups cooked brown rice

Unhidden Valley Ranch Dressing
(page 221) or store-bought vegan
ranch dressing

¼ cup pumpkin seeds

¼ cup thinly sliced scallions

**SERVES 4 · PREP TIME: 10 MINUTES · COOK TIME: 25 MINUTES**

The Cabbage Patch Dance, the Cabbage Patch Kids, and now . . . the Cabbage Patch Bowl! Cabbage has always seemed a forgotten ingredient to me. I look at it and think, "What can you do for me, cabbage?" The truth is that it's very adaptable and goes well with everything! In this recipe I pair it with a couple of my favorite veggies and my all-time favorite dressing. I hope it brings a smile to your face as it does to mine.

**1.** Preheat the oven to 425°F. Line a baking sheet with parchment paper.

**2.** In a large bowl, toss the potato cubes with 1 tablespoon of olive oil, ¼ teaspoon of salt, and ¼ teaspoon of pepper. Spread out on the prepared baking sheet. Bake for 15 minutes.

**3.** While the potatoes are baking, in the same bowl, toss the broccoli and cabbage with the tamari and the remaining 1 tablespoon of olive oil, ¼ teaspoon of salt, and ¼ teaspoon of pepper.

**4.** After the potatoes have baked for 15 minutes, toss them on the baking sheet with a spatula. Add the broccoli and cabbage on top of the potatoes and bake for 10 more minutes, or until the potatoes are fork-tender. Toss the vegetables and potatoes together until well combined.

**5.** Divide the rice among 4 bowls and top with the vegetable mixture. Drizzle with ranch dressing and sprinkle with the pumpkin seeds and scallions.

## VARIATIONS

**CABBAGE PATCH TACOS:** Fill taco shells with the vegetable mixture and top with vegan cheddar shreds, salsa, and Sour Cream (page 222). Chop the broccoli into tiny bits when prepping the ingredients to ensure everything fits nicely inside the taco shells.

**CABBAGE PATCH CHOPPY SALAD:** Prepare all the ingredients as per the recipe, and toss with 1 head romaine lettuce, chopped, and 1 chopped red bell pepper. When everything is combined, chop again for a super-delicious and colorful chopped salad. Top with ranch.

**TIP:** *It is helpful to make a batch of rice or quinoa on a Sunday night so you have it to use throughout the week. It allows you to play around with vegetables and greens a bit, having a cooked grain on hand to add to the mix.*

# Spinach and Mushroom Pizza Bowl

  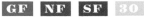 

SERVES 4 • PREP TIME: 10 MINUTES • COOK TIME: 5 MINUTES

1 tablespoon olive oil

1 small yellow bell pepper, seeded and thinly sliced

½ red onion, thinly sliced

1 (8-ounce) package baby bella or white button mushrooms, stemmed and quartered

1 teaspoon Italian seasoning

2 garlic cloves, minced

2 cups Magnificent Marinara (page 231) or store-bought marinara

1 (5-ounce) package baby spinach

2 cups cooked brown rice

1 cup black or kalamata olives, pitted and sliced

Red pepper flakes, for garnish (optional)

Walnut Parmesan (page 230) or store-bought vegan Parmesan, for garnish (optional)

Chopped fresh basil, for garnish (optional)

Pizza is my favorite food from now until the end of time, forever and always. I love any and all variations, and as long as there's sauce and fresh vegetables, I'm a happy man. When I film *The Vegan Roadie* or do television appearances, I like to be conscious and lay off the carbs, but that doesn't mean I'm done with pizza. I came up with this recipe to satisfy my pizza craving when I'm trying to make sure my waistline doesn't expand.

**1.** Heat the oil in a large skillet over medium-high heat. Add the bell pepper, red onion, mushrooms, and Italian seasoning. Sauté for 3 to 5 minutes, until the onion is soft and the mushrooms have reduced in size. Add the garlic and sauté for 1 additional minute, or until fragrant.

**2.** Spoon ¼ cup of marinara sauce into each of 4 bowls. Top with the spinach, followed by the rice and sautéed vegetables. Top each bowl with the remaining sauce and the olives.

**3.** Garnish with red pepper flakes, Parmesan, and chopped basil, if desired.

## VARIATIONS

**PIZZA! PIZZA!** Omit the rice and make this an actual pizza! Generously brush your favorite store-bought vegan crust with olive oil, top with marinara, spinach, and sautéed vegetables, and drizzle with Easy Cheese Sauce–Mozzarella variation (page 224) or store-bought vegan mozzarella shreds. Bake at 375°F for 12 to 15 minutes, until the edges of the crust start to brown. Garnish with red pepper flakes, Walnut Parmesan, and fresh basil, if desired.

**PIZZA BOWL DELUXE:** Add your favorite vegan Italian sausage, cut into bite-size pieces, and top with Easy Cheese Sauce–Mozzarella variation (page 224) or store-bought vegan mozzarella shreds.

**TIP:** *Top off any veggie bowl like this with some chia seeds or hemp seeds for extra protein.*

# Kale and Sweet Potato Hash

**GF** **NF** **SF**

2 tablespoons olive oil

1 onion, chopped

2 garlic cloves, minced

2 medium sweet potatoes, peeled and cut into ½-inch cubes

1 teaspoon smoked paprika

1 teaspoon dried rosemary

½ cup low-sodium vegetable broth

1 large bunch curly kale, stemmed and roughly chopped (about 4 cups)

½ teaspoon sea salt

¼ teaspoon black pepper

**SERVES 4 • PREP TIME: 15 MINUTES • COOK TIME: 25 MINUTES**

Kale is at its finest when combined with something everyone swoons over, like sweet potatoes. I have mentioned already that the struggle is real when getting greens on the plate. This hash is just another way that I love to sneak them in! Not to mention it totally works as a breakfast food.

**1.** Heat the oil in a large skillet over medium heat. Add the onion and sauté for 3 minutes, or until soft. Add the garlic and sauté for 1 additional minute, or until fragrant.

**2.** Add the potatoes, smoked paprika, and rosemary to the skillet. Mix well to combine and sauté for 5 minutes, or until the potatoes are just barely starting to brown.

**3.** Slowly stir in the broth, being careful as it will spatter. Cover and simmer for 7 minutes; the liquid should be bubbling.

**4.** Add the kale on top of the potatoes and cover again. Continue to simmer for 2 minutes, or until the kale is wilted. Add the salt and pepper and mix well to combine. Continue to simmer, uncovered, for 5 minutes, or until the liquid has evaporated and the potatoes are fork-tender.

### VARIATIONS

**BREAKFAST PLATTER:** Top with Scrappy Scrambler (page 138) for a complete breakfast.

**WESTERN SKILLET:** Dice up 1 jalapeño pepper and 1 red bell pepper to make this a Western skillet with a kick. Add the peppers when adding the garlic.

**TIP:** *You can prep the sweet potatoes ahead of time if you are planning a gathering for a brunch. Peel and cube the potatoes and submerge them in cold water. Cover and store in the refrigerator for up to 2 days before cooking.*

# Shaved Cabbage and Brussels Sprouts with Mustard Sauce

GF  NF  30

¼ cup Mayonnaise (page 223) or store-bought vegan mayonnaise

2 tablespoons whole-grain mustard

1 tablespoon olive oil

1 pound Brussels sprouts, trimmed and thinly sliced (about 2 cups)

1 teaspoon sea salt

1 teaspoon black pepper

2 cups thinly sliced green cabbage (about ¼ head)

SERVES 4 • PREP TIME: 10 MINUTES • COOK TIME: 10 MINUTES

What's the strongest vegetable? A muscle sprout! No, but really, Brussels sprouts are packed full of vitamins and nutrients. They're also that vegetable people secretly love. If you are still screaming that you dislike them, try this recipe with its quick sauce to see if it changes your mind!

**1.** In a small bowl, mix the mayonnaise and mustard. Set aside.

**2.** In a large skillet, heat the oil over medium-high heat. Add the Brussels sprouts, salt, and pepper and sear on each side for 2 minutes. Lower the heat to medium, add the cabbage, and cook for 2 to 4 minutes, until just tender.

**3.** Divide among 4 plates and drizzle with the mustard sauce.

### VARIATIONS

**CABBAGE AND BRUSSELS BOWL:** Add 1 (8-ounce) package baby bella or white button mushrooms, stemmed and sliced, for a heartier texture. Sauté them for 2 minutes, then add the Brussels sprouts and continue with the recipe as written. Fill your bowls with brown rice or quinoa and top with this recipe.

**FANCY CABBAGE AND BRUSSELS SUB SANDWICH:** Toss this mixture on a hoagie with some Basic Baked Tofu (page 137) for a hearty sandwich.

**TIP:** Shave the Brussels sprouts and cabbage with the slicing blade on a food processor or mandoline. If you don't have either, don't stress it. Just use a sharp knife to slice them as thin as you can for the same results.

# Savory Cabbage and Scallion Pancakes with Spicy Peanut Dipping Sauce

SERVES 4 • PREP TIME: 10 MINUTES • COOK TIME: 15 MINUTES

**FOR THE DIPPING SAUCE**

¼ cup creamy peanut butter

¼ cup water

2 teaspoons soy sauce or gluten-free tamari

1 teaspoon sriracha sauce

**FOR THE PANCAKES**

1 cup all-purpose flour

1 tablespoon baking powder

1¼ cups low-sodium vegetable broth

1 tablespoon soy sauce or gluten-free tamari

2 cups shredded green cabbage

6 scallions (both white and green parts), thinly sliced

2 garlic cloves, minced

½ teaspoon sea salt

¼ teaspoon black pepper

1 tablespoon olive oil, plus more as needed

I love old-school scallion pancakes! But I also love cabbage and have been on a constant quest to find delicious ways to work more veggies into my life. I had friends over for a round of taste-testing for this book, and this recipe received the highest marks all around. I hope it's a smash with your friends, too!

**1.** *To make the dipping sauce:* In a small bowl, whisk together the peanut butter, water, soy sauce, and sriracha until well combined. Set aside.

**2.** *To make the pancakes:* In a large bowl, whisk together the flour, baking powder, broth, and soy sauce. Fold in the cabbage, scallions, garlic, salt, and pepper.

**3.** Heat 1 tablespoon of oil in a medium skillet over medium-high heat. For each pancake, pour ½ cup of batter into the skillet. When small bubbles appear in the center of the pancake, flip it and flatten it with the back of a spatula. Let it cook on the other side until lightly browned and cooked through, 1 to 2 more minutes.

**4.** Repeat with the remaining batter, adding more oil to the skillet as needed.

**5.** Cut the pancakes into quarters and serve with the peanut sauce on the side for dipping.

**VARIATIONS**

**MANGO SCALLION PANCAKES:** Replace the cabbage with 2 cups finely chopped mango.

**APP AND ENTRÉE PLATE:** Serve this dish alongside Stan's Cauliflower Fried Rice (page 112) for a complete meal.

**TIP:** *If peanut butter isn't your thing, use any nut butter that you love for the dipping sauce. What's important is that your finished sauce is creamy, sweet, savory, and a touch spicy. If needed, add more water by the teaspoon to reach the desired consistency.*

# Ethiopian Cabbage, Carrot, and Potato Stew

   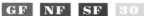

**GF** **NF** **SF** **30**

3 russet potatoes, peeled and cut into ½-inch cubes

2 tablespoons olive oil

6 carrots, peeled, halved lengthwise, and cut into ½-inch slices

1 onion, chopped

4 garlic cloves, minced

1 tablespoon ground turmeric

1 teaspoon ground cumin

1 teaspoon ground ginger

1½ teaspoons sea salt

1½ cups low-sodium vegetable broth, divided

4 cups shredded or thinly sliced green cabbage

SERVES 4 TO 6 • PREP TIME: 10 MINUTES •
COOK TIME: 20 MINUTES

Properly known as *atakilt wat*, this incredibly tasty stew is surprisingly simple to make. I have not had the opportunity to enjoy Ethiopian food as much as I would like, but I can say that each time has been a delightful experience. It's fun to sit around a plate with friends and share a meal, too! Some of my favorite Ethiopian restaurants I have found on my travels are Bunna Cafe (Brooklyn, New York), Blue Nile Cafe (Kansas City, Missouri), and Blue Nile Ethiopian Kitchen (Memphis, Tennessee). I hope you can check them out if you ever find yourself in those parts.

**1.** Bring a large pot of water to a boil over medium-high heat. Add the potatoes and cook for 10 minutes, or until fork-tender. Drain and set aside.

**2.** While the potatoes are cooking, heat the oil in a large skillet over medium-high heat. Add the carrots and onion and sauté for 5 minutes. Add the garlic, turmeric, cumin, ginger, and salt and sauté for 1 additional minute, until fragrant.

**3.** Add the cooked potatoes and 1 cup of broth to the skillet, bring to a boil, and reduce to a simmer. Scatter the cabbage on top of the potatoes. Cover and simmer for 3 minutes.

**4.** Mix the cabbage into the potatoes, add the remaining ½ cup of broth, cover, and simmer for 5 more minutes, or until the cabbage is wilted and tender. Stir the cabbage from time to time while cooking to incorporate it with the other ingredients as it continues to wilt.

## VARIATIONS

**ETHIOPIAN PITA:** Serve this inside a pita with chopped spinach and brown rice. Drizzle with sriracha, if desired.

**GREEN STEW:** Use 2 cups of cabbage instead of 4 cups. After the cabbage has mostly wilted down, add 2 cups roughly chopped kale and simmer for 2 to 4 more minutes to allow the kale to wilt down. Stir into the stew until well incorporated.

**TIP:** *Make this on a Sunday night for a bunch of mix-and-match meals through the week. It pairs nicely with almost any green or grain for a complete meal.*

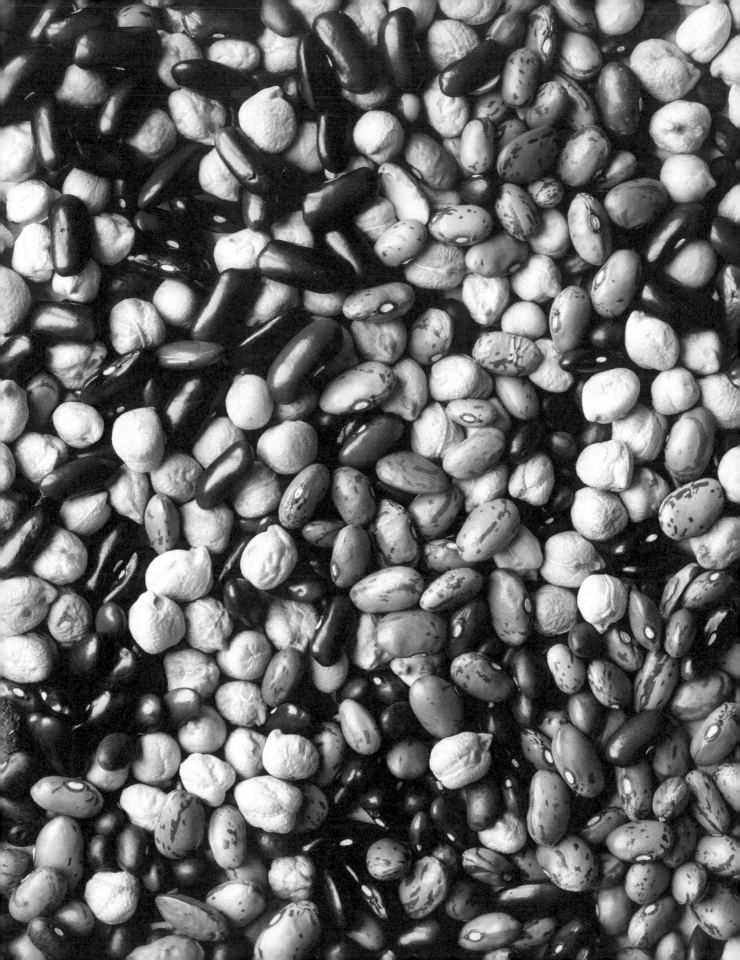

# CHAPTER 3

# Beans

Beans are extremely versatile and good for us in many ways. Pretty much all beans are excellent sources of protein and fiber. They are naturally fat-free, sodium-free, and cholesterol-free. Many types are also good sources of potassium. There are so many types to choose from, too: black, great northern, cannellini, kidney, navy, pink, pinto, and on and on. Not convinced yet? Then leave all the facts out of it and instead focus on this chapter full of delicious recipes that prove just how versatile, scrumptious, and easy beans can be.

Within these pages, I'm going to stick to beans that are probably familiar to you. Most of the recipes in this chapter call for beans from a can, for the plain and simple reason that beans from a can are easy. Again, I'm committed to the "simple" promise of this book. When buying, I always look for beans in cans free of BPA.

But dried beans don't always have to be difficult, and they are cheaper, so I'm giving you recipes that use both. Along with that, I'm also going to start you off with a basic dried-bean cooking method, so you can make batches of beans to build fresh versions of the GGB Bowl (page 28) whenever you want. If you find you prefer dried beans, by all means, feel free to substitute 1½ cups cooked dried beans whenever a recipe calls for 1 (15-ounce) can of beans.

# THE BASICS OF COOKING BEANS

Cooking dried beans from scratch is simple, and you can save time by cooking large batches and freezing the extras in portioned amounts.

You have two soaking options—an overnight soak or a quick soak—but by all means, soak your beans if you're making a straightforward batch of beans. Soaking beans makes them cook faster. It's also thought that soaking the beans aids in breaking down some of the complex sugars that can make beans hard for some people to digest. However, I'm not offering any guarantees on digestibility because every stomach is different.

## TO SOAK THE BEANS

Before soaking beans, be sure to rinse them thoroughly and sift through them with your fingers. Discard any beans that are shriveled, broken, undersized, or discolored, as well as any pebbles, stones, or debris.

*For overnight soaking:* Empty a 1-pound bag of dried beans into a large stockpot and add cool water to 2 inches above the level of the beans. Cover and let soak at room temperature for 8 hours or overnight. Do not drain.

*For a quick soak:* Empty a 1-pound bag of dried beans into a large stockpot and add cool water to 2 inches above the level of the beans. Cover, bring to a boil, remove from the heat, and let soak for 1 hour. Do not drain.

## TO COOK THE BEANS

Many people choose to cook dried beans in the water they were soaked in, and it is perfectly fine to do so. However, if you are of the camp that wishes to avoid certain undesirable side effects (that's code for gas), then it is key to drain and rinse the beans, and then use fresh water for cooking.

**1.** Add 1½ teaspoons sea salt to the water and beans in the stockpot, cover, and bring to a boil over medium heat. Uncover, reduce the heat, and simmer for 1 hour, or until the beans are tender and creamy.

**2.** If you check at 1 hour and the beans are not yet tender, add more water, if necessary, to keep the beans submerged, and cook for another 30 minutes, or until tender and creamy.

**TIP:** *Use the prepared beans in the GGB Bowl (page 28) throughout the week, or in the recipes that follow in this chapter. You can also freeze them in batches. To thaw, remove them from the freezer 1 hour before you begin cooking.*

# White Bean Bruschetta

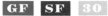

**GF** **SF** **30**

1 (15-ounce) can cannellini beans, rinsed and drained

3 plum tomatoes, seeded and chopped

1 garlic clove, minced

¼ cup chopped pitted kalamata olives

2 tablespoons olive oil

¼ cup chopped fresh basil

¼ teaspoon sea salt

¼ teaspoon black pepper

1 baguette, sliced ½ inch thick and toasted

**SERVES 4 TO 6 • PREP TIME: 10 MINUTES**

This appetizer is quick and easy to put together, but your guests will think you went to a lot of trouble when they take a bite! Loaded with flavor, it always has my friends oohing and aahing—and yours will, too!

**1.** In a large bowl, combine the beans, tomatoes, garlic, olives, oil, basil, salt, and pepper. Mix together until well combined.

**2.** Dollop a heaping tablespoon onto each toasted baguette slice and serve on an appetizer platter.

### VARIATIONS

**CALIFORNIA BRUSCHETTA:** Replace the beans and olives with 2 avocados (peeled, pitted, and diced) and ¼ cup minced red onion. Add 1 teaspoon balsamic vinegar and top with Walnut Parmesan (page 230).

**ENDIVE BRUSCHETTA BOATS:** Use endive leaves instead of bread to cut down on the carbs, and serve with the main recipe or the variation above—or both, for variety!

**TIP:** *Brush your sliced baguette pieces with olive oil and broil for just a minute to achieve a quick toast on several slices at once. Keep an eye on them, as all broilers are different—bread can go from perfectly crisp to burnt in a matter of seconds.*

# White Bean Hummus

 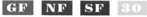  

**GF** **NF** **SF** **30**

1 (15-ounce) can cannellini beans, rinsed and drained

2 tablespoons toasted sesame oil

1 to 3 tablespoons water

1 teaspoon garlic powder

½ teaspoon ground cumin

¼ teaspoon sea salt

¼ teaspoon black pepper

Olive oil, for drizzling

SERVES 6 TO 8 · PREP TIME: 5 MINUTES

Hummus is so versatile! It's typically made with chickpeas, but I put my white-bean version in this book because it is the most blender-friendly. Try this recipe just as it is, or skip ahead to the variations. The Everything Hummus variation is my favorite; I love putting it on a plain toasted vegan bagel.

**1.** Combine the beans, sesame oil, 1 tablespoon of water, garlic powder, cumin, salt, and pepper in a blender and blend until smooth. Add up to 2 tablespoons more water if necessary to achieve the proper consistency.

**2.** Transfer to a serving bowl and drizzle with oil.

### VARIATIONS

**EVERYTHING HUMMUS:** I love everything bagels, so I came up with this variation to dip chips or veggies in and get my "everything" fix. Simply combine 1 tablespoon dried minced onion, 1 tablespoon sesame seeds, 1 teaspoon poppy seeds, 1 teaspoon flaked sea salt, and ¼ teaspoon freshly ground black pepper in a small bowl and sprinkle on top of the hummus.

**PESTO HUMMUS:** Add 2 tablespoons nutritional yeast and ½ cup roughly chopped fresh basil to the blender. You may need to add more water during blending.

**TIP:** *Food processors and high-speed blenders are best for making hummus. You can still use a standard blender, but know that you will have to add more liquid, and the final result won't be a thick hummus, although it will still be delicious.*

# Pinto Bean Queso

GF 30

1 (15-ounce) can pinto beans, rinsed and drained

½ cup chopped onion

2 garlic cloves, minced

1 (5-ounce) can diced green chiles

¼ teaspoon sea salt

¼ teaspoon black pepper

1 cup Easy Cheese Sauce–Queso variation (page 224)

Tortilla chips, for serving (optional)

SERVES 6 TO 8 • PREP TIME: 5 MINUTES • COOK TIME: 25 MINUTES

I was an actor well into my twenties, and cast parties were always full of terrible junk food that was fun, quick, and easy to throw together. A dip that always made the rounds and was devoured had refried beans, cream cheese, and shreds upon shreds of processed dairy cheese. This is my version of that dip—it tastes better and is a whole heck of a lot better for you!

1. Preheat the oven to 400°F.

2. In a large bowl, mash the beans. Add the onion, garlic, chiles with their juice, salt, and pepper and mix well to combine.

3. Transfer the mixture to a 1-quart shallow baking dish and top with the queso. Bake for 25 minutes, or until bubbling.

4. Serve with tortilla chips, if desired.

**VARIATIONS**

**DELUXE PINTO BEAN DIP:** After the dish is baked, drizzle some Sour Cream (page 222) on top and add sliced black olives and thinly sliced scallions to delight the eyes and bellies of your guests.

**BEAN AND CHEESE BURRITOS:** Spoon ½ cup of this recipe onto a 10-inch flour tortilla with a few dashes of hot sauce, roll it up, and enjoy. If you want to thicken it up, add ¼ to ½ cup cooked rice to each burrito.

**TIP:** *If you don't feel like making the vegan queso from this book or you just ran out of raw cashews, top off the pinto mixture with 1 (14.5-ounce) can of diced tomatoes, drained, and store-bought vegan pepper Jack shreds.*

# Black Bean Layer Dip

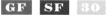 **GF** **SF** **30**

1 (15-ounce) can black beans, rinsed and drained

¼ teaspoon sea salt

¼ teaspoon black pepper

1 cup Sour Cream (page 222) or store-bought vegan sour cream

2 teaspoons Taco Seasoning (page 219) or store-bought taco seasoning

2 medium avocados, peeled, pitted, and mashed

1 cup salsa

1 cup shredded romaine lettuce

2 scallions, chopped

Tortilla chips, for serving

**SERVES 12 · PREP TIME: 15 MINUTES**

Are you always that person at the party with a plate full of hummus and carrots? Bring this dip to the table and you will be bringing the party with you! This is a guaranteed crowd pleaser and "Oh my gosh, that's vegan?!" dish to pass at any occasion.

**1.** In a medium bowl, mash the beans with the salt and pepper.

**2.** In a small bowl, mix the sour cream and taco seasoning.

**3.** Layer all the ingredients in a 1-quart serving dish in the following order: black-bean mixture, sour-cream mixture, avocado, salsa, romaine lettuce, and scallions.

**4.** Scoop up this dip with your favorite tortilla chips!

## VARIATIONS

**SIX-LAYER BURRITOS:** Portion the ingredients to make 12 average-size burritos or 6 monster-size burritos. Roll up the ingredients in an appropriate-size tortilla, put it in your lunch box, and make all your friends jealous.

**SEVEN-LAYER BLACK BEAN DIP:** Add 1 cup Easy Cheese Sauce–Nacho variation (page 224) on top of the avocado layer, then top with the salsa, romaine, and scallions.

**TIP:** *Vegan refried black beans are available, but they are not always easy to find. If they are available, use them in place of the black-bean mixture for easier preparation.*

# Roasted Chickpea and Brussels Sprouts Salad

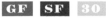 **GF** **SF** 30

1 pound Brussels sprouts, trimmed
   and thinly sliced

1 (15-ounce) can chickpeas, rinsed
   and drained

2 tablespoons olive oil

Juice of 1 lemon

¾ teaspoon sea salt

¾ teaspoon black pepper

⅓ cup roughly chopped walnuts

Walnut Parmesan (page 230) or
   store-bought vegan Parmesan,
   for garnish

**SERVES 4 • PREP TIME: 5 MINUTES • COOK TIME: 25 MINUTES**

Brussels sprouts get a bad rep, but people love chickpeas. I happen to love both, so I combined the two in the oven to get a crispy finish that serves up nicely as a side dish or even the main event. It's no muss, no fuss, with everything on one pan—perfect for a quick dinner. Don't forget to pat those chickpeas dry with a paper towel after they are rinsed and drained, so they crisp up nicely when roasted.

**1.** Preheat the oven to 400°F. Line a baking sheet with parchment paper.

**2.** In a large bowl, toss the Brussels sprouts and chickpeas with the oil, lemon juice, salt, and pepper. Spread the mixture on the prepared baking sheet and roast for 15 minutes. Add the walnuts and toss the mixture. Roast for another 10 minutes.

**3.** Serve warm, garnished with Parmesan.

**VARIATIONS**

**SOUTHWEST CHICKPEA AND BRUSSELS SALAD:** For a Southwest flair, roast 1 cup corn kernels and 1 red bell pepper, seeded and chopped, with the Brussels sprouts and chickpeas.

**ROASTED CHICKPEA AND BRUSSELS BOWL:** Make this a meal by adding a kale base mixed with chopped tomatoes and cucumbers and topped with pepitas (roasted pumpkin seeds) for an extra crunch. Drizzle on the dressing of your choice.

**TIP:** *Using packaged Brussels sprouts that have already been trimmed and sliced is a great time saver, if you can get your hands on them!*

# Pinto, Corn, and Avocado Salad

 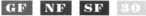  

**GF** **NF** **SF** **30**

1 (15-ounce) can pinto beans, rinsed and drained

1 cup cherry tomatoes, halved

1½ cups frozen (and thawed) or fresh corn kernels

1 avocado, peeled, pitted, and diced

¼ cup chopped fresh cilantro

Juice of 1 lime

1 tablespoon maple syrup or agave

1 tablespoon olive oil

¾ teaspoon sea salt

½ teaspoon black pepper

SERVES 4 • PREP TIME: 10 MINUTES

I'm not a fan of your standard bean salad, so I wanted to spruce this up a bit for an easy go-to salad to make for lunches midweek. This one is truly simple and, most importantly, delicious. Enjoy mixing and matching this with greens and grains for a full vegan plate.

**1.** In a large bowl, mix the beans, tomatoes, corn, avocado, and cilantro until well combined.

**2.** Add the lime juice, maple syrup, oil, salt, and pepper and stir until all ingredients are evenly coated.

**3.** Serve immediately or chill before serving.

### VARIATIONS

**PINTO, CORN, AND AVOCADO BOWL:** Make it a bowl! Start with a layer of chopped romaine lettuce, add brown rice, then top with a serving of this recipe.

**PINTO, CORN, AND AVOCADO WRAP:** Add Basic Baked Tofu (page 137), your green of choice, and a serving of this recipe to a 10-inch flour tortilla and roll it up for a great lunch on the go!

**TIP:** *Hold off on adding the avocado and let the salad sit, covered, in the refrigerator for a couple of hours or overnight before serving, and the flavors will become more prominent. Add the avocado just before serving.*

# Black Bean, Cucumber, and Feta Salad

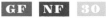

1 (15-ounce) can black beans, rinsed and drained

1 cucumber, peeled and diced

1 recipe Fast Feta (page 225)

SERVES 6 • PREP TIME: 5 MINUTES

Refreshing and full of protein, the feta in this salad adds a Greek twist to ingredients that aren't typically used together for a delicious surprise! Requiring very little prep and no cooking, this is a versatile go-to summer dish—serve it over lettuce, scoop it up with corn chips, or even toss it into a wrap for a quick meal on the go.

In a large bowl, toss together all the ingredients. Serve immediately or chill before serving.

### VARIATIONS

**REFRESHING BLACK BEAN, CUCUMBER, AND FAST FETA SALAD:** For a refreshing touch, add 2 tablespoons minced fresh mint.

**BLACK BEAN, CUCUMBER, AND FETA BOWL:** Add this to a bowl of massaged kale and brown rice for a complete meal. If you toss it all together, the feta gives the entire bowl just enough flavor, no dressing required. If you feel it's dry, add a squeeze of lime juice.

**TIP:** *If time allows, let this chill overnight. All the seasoning on the feta will settle in with the rest of the dish and make a great flavor profile the next day.*

# White and Green Beans with Browned Butter

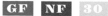

¼ cup vegan butter

3 garlic cloves, thinly sliced

1 pound green beans, trimmed and halved

1 (15-ounce) can cannellini beans, rinsed and drained

2 pinches sea salt

¼ teaspoon black pepper

Walnut Parmesan (page 230) or store-bought vegan Parmesan, for garnish (optional)

**SERVES 4 • PREP TIME: 5 MINUTES • COOK TIME: 10 MINUTES**

Green beans are a classic, but adding some white beans to the mix with the browned butter gives it a special touch, don't you think? This is the perfect side dish for any meal and also a great recipe to serve up at a holiday meal.

**1.** Melt the butter in a large skillet over medium–high heat for 3 to 5 minutes, until it begins to brown and smell nutty. Lower the heat to medium, add the garlic, and sauté for 15 to 30 seconds, until just fragrant. Be careful not to let it burn.

**2.** Add the green beans and sauté for 3 minutes, or until seared, stirring frequently to keep the garlic from burning (a little browning is okay).

**3.** Add the cannellini beans, salt, and pepper and cook for an additional 2 minutes, or until heated through.

**4.** Serve hot, garnished with the Parmesan, if desired.

**VARIATIONS**

**GREEN BEANS AND RED GRAPES:** Replace the butter with 2 tablespoons olive oil. Replace the white beans with 1 cup halved seedless red grapes. Sauté for 5 minutes, or until the grapes are fork-tender.

**GREEN BEANS ALMANDINE:** Replace the white beans with 1 cup slivered almonds.

**TIP:** *Fresh green beans taste the best in this recipe and hold a nice crunch. But you can use frozen green beans without having to worry about trimming and chopping in half.*

# Slow-Cooker Black Bean Taco Chili

**GF** **NF** **SF**

1 (1-pound) bag dried black beans

1 onion, chopped

3 garlic cloves, minced

1 green bell pepper, seeded and diced

1½ cups frozen corn kernels

3 tablespoons Taco Seasoning
(page 219) or store-bought taco
seasoning

4 cups low-sodium vegetable broth

1 (28-ounce) can diced tomatoes

1 teaspoon sea salt

Chopped fresh cilantro, for garnish
(optional)

Vegan cheddar shreds, for garnish
(optional)

Sour Cream (page 222) or
store-bought vegan sour cream,
for garnish (optional)

**SERVES 8 · PREP TIME: 5 MINUTES · COOK TIME: 8 HOURS**

Anything involving the word "taco" that requires just
tossing the ingredients into a pot and walking away is my
kind of recipe. Chili and tacos collide with this set-and-
forget recipe that will get you through the week or serve a
hungry family on a cold winter night.

**1.** Combine the beans, onion, garlic, bell pepper, corn,
taco seasoning, broth, tomatoes, and salt in a slow cooker.
Cover, and cook on low for 8 hours.

**2.** If needed, season with more salt, to taste.

**3.** Serve hot, garnished with cilantro, cheese, and sour
cream, if desired.

## VARIATIONS

**MEATY TACO CHILI:** Add 1 (12-ounce) package frozen
vegan beef crumbles for the last hour of cooking. If the chili
has already cooked for 8 hours and you want to add the
meat when you get home from work, that's fine. Just add
the crumbles and let them cook on high for 15 minutes.

**TRADITIONAL CHILI:** Replace the black beans with red kidney
beans. Replace the taco seasoning with 2 tablespoons chili
powder. You may have to adjust the seasoning after the
chili has cooked.

**TIP:** *If you're using a slow cooker, you don't have to soak
the beans ahead of time, since they are essentially soaking
for some time as well as cooking. But if you want to soak
them to reduce the likelihood of experiencing gas, go for it!*

**NO SLOW COOKER? NO PROBLEM:** *To prepare this recipe on the
stove, heat 1 tablespoon olive oil in a stockpot over medium
heat. Add the onion and garlic and sauté for 2 minutes, until
fragrant. Add all of the ingredients through sea salt. Cover
and simmer for 1 hour and 30 minutes, until the beans are
tender but not mushy or falling apart. Serve hot with the
toppings, if desired.*

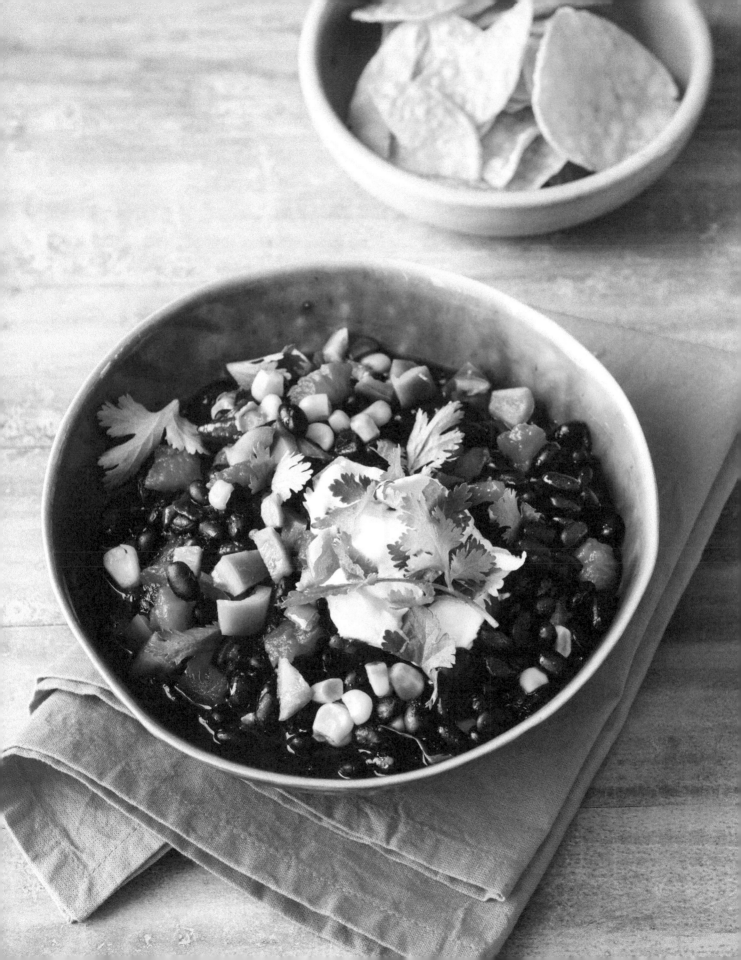

# Slow-Cooker Tuscan White Bean Soup

**GF** **NF** **SF**

1 (1-pound) bag dried great
   northern beans

1 onion, chopped

6 garlic cloves, minced

2 carrots, peeled, halved lengthwise,
   and thinly sliced

3 celery stalks, thinly sliced

8 cups low-sodium vegetable broth

5 fresh rosemary sprigs

2 bay leaves

½ teaspoon salt

½ teaspoon black pepper

¼ teaspoon red pepper flakes

1 (28-ounce) can diced tomatoes

**SERVES 6 TO 8 • PREP TIME: 10 MINUTES • COOK TIME: 8 HOURS**

Nothing makes me nostalgic for a Michigan autumn faster than walking into a home filled with the aroma of a slow cooker that has been chugging away for hours. What a treat to leave for work and return home to a meal! This recipe is just right for sitting around the table for a family meal on a crisp fall evening.

**1.** Combine the beans, onion, garlic, carrots, celery, broth, rosemary, and bay leaves in a slow cooker. Stir well to combine, cover, and cook on low for 8 hours.

**2.** Stir in the salt, black pepper, red pepper flakes, and tomatoes with their juice, cover, and cook on high for 30 minutes.

**3.** Remove the bay leaves and any rosemary sprigs that are still intact, and serve.

### VARIATIONS

**WHITE BEAN AND CORN CHOWDER:** Instead of the tomatoes, stir in 2 cups frozen corn kernels, cover, and cook on high for 30 minutes.

**WHITE BEAN STEW:** Add 2 russet potatoes, peeled and cut into 1-inch cubes, with the other ingredients at the beginning. Cover and cook on low for 8 hours. Then stir in 1 (10-ounce) package baby spinach with the tomatoes, cover, and cook on high for 30 minutes. If necessary, add the spinach in two batches and stir it in as it wilts.

**TIP:** *This recipe was timed and tested at 8 hours cooking time, so you can leave for work and come home to dinner! But if you need it to cook faster, you can cook on high for 4 hours instead.*

**NO SLOW COOKER? NO PROBLEM:** *To prepare this recipe on the stove, heat 1 tablespoon olive oil in a stockpot over medium heat. Add the onion and garlic and sauté for 2 minutes, or until fragrant. Add the remaining ingredients except for the tomatoes, cover, and simmer for 50 to 60 minutes. Add the tomatoes with their juice and cook just until heated through.*

# Chickpea-of-the-Sea Sandwich

 **NF** **30**

1 (15-ounce) can chickpeas, rinsed and drained

¼ cup Mayonnaise (page 223) or store-bought vegan mayonnaise

1 celery stalk, halved and thinly sliced

2 tablespoons minced red onion

1 tablespoon capers, minced

1 teaspoon caper juice

¼ teaspoon sea salt

½ teaspoon black pepper

4 slices vegan bread, toasted

SERVES 2 • PREP TIME: 10 MINUTES

My first memory of a tuna sandwich was my first kiss in the first grade. Lisa Vieau and I were sitting next to each other eating our lunch and she came at me to kiss me with a face full of tuna sandwich. I'm not sure if that aggressive memory is the reason I stayed away from tuna sandwiches for so long, but after I went vegan I became obsessed with the chickpea version and have been perfecting it for years. I hope you enjoy this version—but please, don't kiss anybody while you are eating it.

**1.** In a large bowl, mash the chickpeas with the mayonnaise, celery, red onion, capers, caper juice, salt, and pepper.

**2.** Divide the chickpea mixture between 2 slices of toasted bread and top with the remaining 2 slices of bread. Cut each sandwich in half.

**VARIATIONS**

**CHICKPEA MELT:** Use vegan cheese slices or Easy Cheese Sauce (page 224), tomato slices, and avocado slices to make a truly terrific melt. A trick to melting store-bought vegan sliced cheese: I suggest building the sandwich and heating it in a skillet, covered, over medium-low heat. The heat trapped in the skillet will melt the cheese. Just be sure not to burn the bottom of your sandwich!

**CHICKPEA PASTA SALAD:** Mix this with 3 cups cooked and cooled pasta for a terrific pasta salad. Add a little more mayonnaise, if desired, so the pasta isn't dry.

**TIP:** *Jars of capers are usually small and hard to get a measuring spoon into. I suggest dumping the entire contents into a small bowl, measuring out what you need, and returning the capers and juice to the jar so you don't lose any of the juice!*

# Garlicky BBQ White Bean and Kale Quesadillas

1 (15-ounce) can cannellini beans, rinsed and drained

¼ cup low-sodium vegetable broth

2 tablespoons plus 1 teaspoon olive oil, plus more as needed, divided

Juice of ½ lemon

2 garlic cloves, roughly chopped

½ teaspoon dried rosemary

½ teaspoon sea salt

½ teaspoon black pepper

1 cup stemmed and roughly chopped kale

4 (10-inch) whole-wheat tortillas

Basic BBQ Sauce (page 232) or store-bought vegan barbecue sauce, for serving

**SERVES 4 • PREP TIME: 10 MINUTES • COOK TIME: 15 MINUTES**

Whether served as a meal or an appetizer, this incredibly flavorful and easy bean quesadilla is very difficult for me to share. You have been warned!

1. In a blender, combine the beans, broth, 1 tablespoon of olive oil, lemon juice, garlic, rosemary, salt, and pepper and blend for 1 minute, or until smooth.

2. In a bowl, massage the kale with 1 teaspoon of olive oil for 1 minute, or until soft.

3. Heat the remaining 1 tablespoon of olive oil in a large skillet over medium heat. Place 1 tortilla in the skillet and spread half of the bean mixture on one half of the tortilla, then top with ¼ cup of the kale. Fold the tortilla in half, press down, and cook for 2 minutes on each side, or until golden brown. Repeat with the remaining tortillas and filling ingredients, adding more oil to the pan if needed.

4. Cut each tortilla in quarters and either drizzle with BBQ sauce or serve the sauce on the side.

## VARIATIONS

**WHITE BEAN AND KALE FLATBREAD:** Brush 4 whole-wheat pitas with olive oil and top with the bean purée and kale. Drizzle with BBQ sauce and bake at 350°F for 15 minutes, or until the pitas start to brown at the edges.

**SAY CHEESE QUESADILLA:** Add vegan mozzarella shreds to this quesadilla to give it that extra touch of stretchy, cheesy goodness.

**TIP:** *Blenders vary in speed and ability. Add extra liquid to get this purée going in your blender, if necessary. Start by adding 1 teaspoon olive oil at a time until it starts moving, but be careful not to overdo it as you still want a thick consistency for the quesadilla filling.*

# Grilled Stuffed Pinto and Swiss Chard Burritos

 SF 30

1 tablespoon olive oil, plus more for the skillet

1 onion, chopped

2 garlic cloves, minced

1 (15-ounce) can pinto beans, rinsed and drained

4 teaspoons paprika

½ teaspoon sea salt

½ teaspoon black pepper

1 bunch Swiss chard, trimmed and roughly chopped

4 (10-inch) whole-wheat burrito tortillas

2 cups cooked brown rice

2 avocados, peeled, pitted, and sliced

½ cup Sour Cream (page 222) or store-bought vegan sour cream

Salsa, for garnish (optional)

**TIP:** *When rolling up the ingredients in the tortilla, be sure to wrap it tight from the very beginning, as this will ensure you have enough tortilla left to seal all sides as you go.*

**SERVES 8 · PREP TIME: 10 MINUTES · COOK TIME: 20 MINUTES**

I love burritos! I also love sneaking greens into my favorite foods. Once upon a time I was obsessed with the grilled stuffed burrito at Taco Bell. I enjoyed the crunchy outside so much that I set forth replicating it at home in one easy step and, of course, I'm thrilled to share that with you.

**1.** Heat 1 tablespoon of oil over medium heat in a large skillet. Add the onion and sauté for 3 minutes, until soft, then add the garlic and sauté for 1 additional minute, or until fragrant. Add the beans, paprika, salt, and pepper and stir continuously until the bean mixture is heated through, about 3 minutes. Mix in the chard and cook until wilted, about 3 minutes.

**2.** Build each burrito by placing a tortilla on a flat surface in front of you. Starting at the side closest to you, add ¼ cup rice, ¼ cup chard mixture, a few avocado slices, and 1 tablespoon sour cream. Start gently rolling your burrito upward, folding the sides in when you get halfway and continuing until it's completely rolled up and all the sides are sealed.

**3.** Heat 1 teaspoon of oil in a large skillet over medium-low heat. Place the burrito in the skillet, seam-side down, and place a plate on top to weigh it down. After 2 minutes, flip the burrito, being careful to handle the plate with a towel or oven mitt. Place the plate back on the burrito and cook the other side for another 2 minutes, or until brown and crispy. Repeat until all the burritos are finished and crispy on the outside, using more oil if necessary. Garnish with salsa, if desired.

### VARIATIONS

**MONSTER BURRITO:** Go Chipotle style and add vegan chicken or beef strips, plus Guacamole (page 172) and vegan cheddar shreds. This will be harder to roll up, so be conscious of your filling-to-tortilla ratio.

**BURRITO BOWL:** Serve the burrito filling on a bed of chopped romaine lettuce. Top with Guacamole (page 172), hot sauce, and a squeeze of lime.

# Southwest Pinto Bean Burger

NF 30

2 tablespoons flax meal

¼ cup water

2 (15-ounce) cans pinto beans, rinsed and drained

1 cup vegan breadcrumbs

1 to 2 tablespoons soy sauce or gluten-free tamari

1 teaspoon garlic powder

1 teaspoon ground cumin

½ teaspoon sea salt, plus more if needed

1 teaspoon black pepper, plus more if needed

2 tablespoons olive oil, plus more if needed, divided

2 ripe avocados, peeled, pitted, and mashed

6 vegan hamburger buns

1 cup salsa

SERVES 6 • PREP TIME: 10 MINUTES • COOK TIME: 15 MINUTES

Vegan burgers have been my enemy since the day I went vegan (Sunday, April 12, 2009, if anyone is taking notes). The texture usually disappoints me, and those that have a texture I enjoy seem to require an excruciatingly long process to put together. It was my mission here to offer a burger that is both easy and flavorful—and that doesn't crumble out of the bun on that first bite. Success!

1. In a small bowl, whisk together the flax meal and water. Set aside for 5 minutes to thicken.

2. Mash 1 can of beans in a large bowl. Add the second can of beans whole, along with the breadcrumbs, 1 tablespoon of soy sauce, flax-meal mixture, garlic powder, cumin, salt, and pepper. Mix well to combine. If the mixture is extremely dry, add up to 1 more tablespoon soy sauce.

3. Turn out the mixture onto a clean, flat surface and shape into a 6-inch-long log. Gently roll the log to create smooth sides, packing it in at each end after you roll it to keep it at 6 inches. Cut the log into 6 (1-inch-thick) patties; they should be about 3½ inches in diameter.

4. Heat 1 tablespoon of oil in a large skillet over medium-high heat. Add 3 patties and cook for 3 minutes on each side, or until browned and crisp. Use the second tablespoon of oil for the second batch, and more if necessary.

5. Season the mashed avocado with salt and pepper.

6. Build each burger as follows: bottom bun, burger, 2 tablespoons salsa, ¼ cup avocado mash, top bun.

**VARIATIONS**

**PIZZA BURGER:** I finagle pizza into any situation I possibly can. Top your burger with Magnificent Marinara (page 231), sautéed mushrooms and onions, and Easy Cheese Sauce–Mozzarella variation (page 224) or store-bought vegan mozzarella shreds. To melt the shreds, put all the toppings on after you flip the burger the first time and place a lid on the skillet so the steam melts the cheese.

**GREEK BURGER:** Start with a layer of fresh baby spinach, then add the burger, sliced green olives, and Fast Feta (page 225).

**TIP:** *Get hands-on. The best way to incorporate all these ingredients is to wash those hands and roll up your sleeves. This can be fun for the family if you have kids who like to get in on the cooking. If you can't find flax meal, grind up flaxseed in a coffee bean grinder.*

# Deconstructed Falafel Bowl

1 (15-ounce) can chickpeas, rinsed and drained

2 tablespoons olive oil, divided

1 tablespoon ground coriander

1 tablespoon ground cumin

2 pinches sea salt

2 pinches black pepper

1 bunch curly kale, stemmed and roughly chopped

1 cup thinly sliced cucumber

1 pint cherry tomatoes, halved

½ red onion, thinly sliced

½ cup roughly chopped fresh cilantro

¼ cup roughly chopped fresh parsley

¼ cup roughly chopped fresh mint

Green Goddess Dressing (page 220) or store-bought vegan green goddess dressing

Pita chips, for serving (optional)

**SERVES 4 · PREP TIME: 20 MINUTES · COOK TIME: 20 MINUTES**

I used to love the tasty falafel from the street carts in New York City. This bowl is in honor of those thrown-together platters, because you can add all these spices to your chickpeas, let them roast for a bit, and then toss it all atop a delicious bowl of veggies—a much healthier option than that street platter! And it just so happens to be vegan.

**1.** Preheat the oven to 425°F. Line a baking sheet with parchment paper.

**2.** In a medium bowl, toss the chickpeas with 1½ tablespoons of olive oil, coriander, cumin, salt, and pepper. Spread on the prepared baking sheet and roast for 10 minutes, toss, and roast for an additional 10 minutes, or until crispy and browned. Remove from the oven and let sit for 5 minutes.

**3.** While the chickpeas are cooling, toss the kale with the remaining ½ tablespoon of olive oil in a large bowl and massage the kale with your hands for 2 minutes, or until soft. Add the cucumber, tomatoes, red onion, cilantro, parsley, and mint. Toss to combine.

**4.** Divide the salad among 4 bowls, top with the chickpeas, and drizzle on the desired amount of dressing. Add the optional pita chips for an extra crunch!

### VARIATIONS

**PROTEIN FALAFEL BOWL:** Add Basic Baked Tofu (page 137) and Quinoa and Broccoli Tabbouleh (page 100) to the bowls and top with chia or hemp seeds for additional protein.

**DECONSTRUCTED FALAFEL PITAS:** Use 4 to 6 whole-wheat pitas (depending on the size of your pita). Drizzle a little dressing inside the pita to start, stuff with everything, and drizzle more dressing on top.

**TIP:** *Chickpeas roast and crisp up better when they are dried thoroughly to start. After they are rinsed and drained, lay them out on a paper towel–lined plate. Add another paper towel on top and gently pat with your hand to absorb all the moisture.*

# Sheet-Pan Black Bean Home Fries

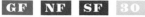 **30**

2 russet potatoes, cut into
½-inch cubes

1 (15-ounce) can black beans, rinsed
and drained

1 red bell pepper, seeded and diced

1 onion, diced

3 tablespoons olive oil

1 teaspoon garlic powder

1 teaspoon chili powder

1 teaspoon ground cumin

¾ teaspoon sea salt

1 teaspoon black pepper

Sour Cream (page 222) or store-bought
vegan sour cream, for garnish
(optional)

Chopped fresh cilantro, for garnish
(optional)

SERVES 4 TO 6 · PREP TIME: 10 MINUTES ·
COOK TIME: 20 MINUTES

I heart potatoes. More specifically, I heart any potato that comes with my breakfast and has the word *home*, *hash*, or *fry* in it. But I mostly love pairing things with my potatoes and throwing them into the oven for an easy mash-up of tasty goodness, and these potatoes with some ketchup hit the spot, every time.

**1.** Preheat the oven to 425°F. Line a baking sheet with parchment paper.

**2.** In a large bowl, combine the potatoes, beans, bell pepper, onion, oil, garlic powder, chili powder, cumin, salt, and black pepper. Toss well to combine.

**3.** Spread the mixture evenly on the prepared baking sheet. Bake for 12 minutes, toss, and bake for an additional 8 minutes, or until the potatoes have turned golden brown and are fork-tender.

**4.** Serve garnished with sour cream and cilantro, if desired.

### VARIATIONS

**SHEET-PAN GARDEN VEGETABLE HOME FRIES:** Replace the beans and bell pepper with sliced zucchini and corn to give this a light summer flair.

**HOME FRY BREAKFAST BOWL:** Combine this with Scrappy Scrambler (page 138) atop a bed of arugula or spinach, drizzled with Garlic-Sriracha Aioli (page 223), for a hearty and nutritious breakfast bowl.

**TIP:** *Ovens vary in their heat. Some might require a few minutes longer for the potatoes to cook all the way through. Test by piercing a piece of potato with a fork. If the fork easily goes all the way in, the potatoes are ready to eat.*

# Swedish Chickpea Balls

1 tablespoon olive oil

2 cups baby bella or white button mushrooms, stemmed and diced

½ cup chopped onion

3 garlic cloves, minced

1 (15-ounce) can chickpeas, rinsed, drained, and mashed

1½ cups vegan breadcrumbs

¼ cup chopped fresh parsley

¼ cup unsweetened applesauce

2 tablespoons soy sauce or gluten-free tamari

½ teaspoon onion powder

½ teaspoon garlic powder

¼ teaspoon paprika

¼ teaspoon caraway seeds

¼ teaspoon fennel seeds

½ teaspoon sea salt

2 pinches cayenne pepper

1 batch Creamy Dreamy Swedish Gravy (page 228)

Minced fresh parsley, for garnish (optional)

**SERVES 4 TO 6 • PREP TIME: 15 MINUTES • COOK TIME: 30 MINUTES**

Don't let this list of ingredients scare you! It is mostly seasonings, and there are only two on the list that may (or may not) be tricky to find: caraway and fennel seeds. If you don't feel like tracking down these two, skip them! But I do encourage you to seek them out, because once you make these chickpea balls, you will want to make them again and again. These are great served over a plate of pasta or all on their own.

**1.** Preheat the oven to 400°F. Line a baking sheet with parchment paper.

**2.** Heat the oil in a large skillet over medium heat. Add the mushrooms and onion. Sauté for 5 minutes, or until the onion is soft and the mushrooms have reduced in size. Add the garlic and cook for 1 additional minute, or until fragrant. Transfer the mixture to a large bowl.

**3.** Add the mashed chickpeas, breadcrumbs, parsley, applesauce, soy sauce, onion powder, garlic powder, paprika, caraway seeds, fennel seeds, salt, and cayenne. Mix the ingredients together; best to roll up your sleeves here and mix everything with your hands to get it well incorporated.

**4.** Scoop out a heaping tablespoon, roll it into a ball with your hands, and place it on the prepared baking sheet. Repeat with the rest of the mixture. Bake for 15 minutes, then turn the balls over. Bake for an additional 10 minutes, or until lightly browned.

**5.** While the meatballs are cooking, gently warm the gravy in a medium saucepan. Add the meatballs to the warm gravy and serve sprinkled with fresh parsley, if desired.

**SPAGHETTI AND MEATBALLS:** Instead of Creamy Dreamy Swedish Gravy, use Magnificent Marinara (page 231) and spaghetti, for a spaghetti meatball dinner.

**MEATBALL MARINARA SUB:** Spoon these meatballs and gravy into a hoagie with sautéed bell peppers, onions, and vegan mayonnaise for the best meatball sandwich ever! Mayo on a meatball sub? I know! An old friend of mine used to do this in high school and I thought it was vile . . . until I tried it one day, and I have never looked back. Be adventurous!

**TIP:** *A drier mixture results in a better texture for these meatballs. If you feel they are too wet when mixing, don't be scared to add a touch more breadcrumbs.*

# Spanish Chickpeas with Tomatoes and Spinach

GF NF SF 30

1 tablespoon olive oil

1 onion, chopped

2 garlic cloves, minced

2 teaspoons ground cumin

2 teaspoons paprika

1 (15-ounce) can chickpeas, rinsed
and drained

1 (14-ounce) can diced tomatoes

⅓ cup raisins

½ teaspoon sea salt

½ teaspoon black pepper

1 (5-ounce) package baby spinach

**SERVES 4 TO 6 • PREP TIME: 5 MINUTES •
COOK TIME: 10 MINUTES**

Something about this one-skillet dish makes my taste buds sing! I love how easily it comes together, and it's the perfect dish to make on a lazy day when you need something delicious and fast.

**1.** Heat the oil in a large skillet over medium heat. Add the onion and sauté for 3 minutes, or until soft. Add the garlic, cumin, and paprika and sauté for 1 additional minute, or until fragrant.

**2.** Add the chickpeas, tomatoes with their juice, raisins, salt, and pepper and mix well to combine. Heat through, about 3 minutes. Add the spinach and mix well to combine; cook until wilted, about 3 minutes.

### VARIATIONS

**GRAINS, GREENS, AND BEANS:** Add this to some rice or quinoa for a complete vegan plate.

**SPANISH CHICKPEA BAKED POTATO:** Cut 2 large russet potatoes in half, rub each half with olive oil, and sprinkle with sea salt. Put the potatoes on a baking sheet and bake at 425°F for 30 minutes, or until fork-tender, flipping once during baking. Top with the chickpea mixture, Sour Cream (page 222), and chopped fresh parsley.

**TIP:** *This is a great recipe to make ahead for the week, because you can eat it as is or make one of the variations above for a complete meal.*

# Chickpea Hush Puppies with Garlic-Sriracha Aioli

**NF** **30**

1 (15-ounce) can chickpeas, rinsed and drained

½ cup minced onion

2 garlic cloves, minced

6 tablespoons unsweetened soy or almond milk

¾ cup yellow cornmeal

½ cup all-purpose flour

2 teaspoons baking powder

1 teaspoon sea salt

Canola oil, for frying

Garlic-Sriracha Aioli (page 223), for serving

SERVES 8 TO 12 • PREP TIME: 10 MINUTES • COOK TIME: 10 MINUTES

Oh, the fast food of it all! I want you to be a healthy and happy person. I firmly believe that means finding a balance. This is the only recipe in the book that calls for you to actually fry something. Below, in the Tip, I have included a baked version if you have to have these but can't imagine frying (I get that and support it). Just the same, it's a treat, and we all want a treat now and then. If you don't want to make the aioli, serve the hush puppies as I often do: with straight-up ketchup.

**1.** In a large bowl, mash the chickpeas with the onion, garlic, milk, cornmeal, flour, baking powder, and salt. Mix until well combined.

**2.** Pour about 2 inches of oil into a heavy, deep skillet or saucepot. Heat the oil to 350°F; when it's at the right temperature, a drop of batter will sizzle when added.

**3.** While the oil is heating, take a heaping teaspoon for each hush puppy and roll it into a ball, then set it aside on a plate.

**4.** When the oil reaches temperature, use a slotted spoon to slide the hush puppies, in batches, into the hot oil. Fry until golden brown, 1 to 2 minutes, then transfer to a paper towel–lined plate.

**5.** Serve with the aioli.

**VARIATIONS**

**OKRA HUSH PUPPIES:** Mix ½ cup chopped frozen (and thawed) okra into the batter.

**JALAPEÑO POPPER HUSH PUPPIES:** Mix 1 minced jalapeño pepper into the batter.

**TIP:** *Make a more healthful version of these by baking them on a parchment-lined baking sheet at 425°F for 10 minutes. Flip and bake for 8 more minutes, until golden brown.*

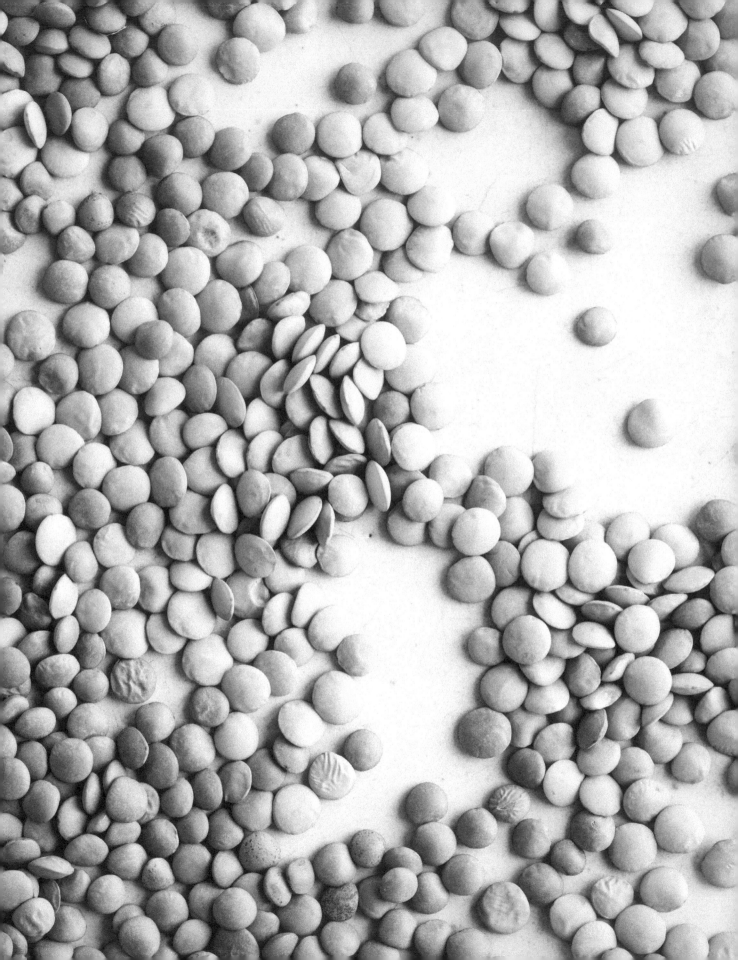

# CHAPTER 4

# Lentils

Cooking lentils is as easy as rinse, simmer, and serve! There are a variety of lentils that can be cooked a myriad of ways, and the preparation is always simple. This chapter includes recipes using dried lentils, as well as some using canned lentils for convenience.

And here we are with protein again: Cooked lentils provide 18 grams of protein per cup, for yet another way to effortlessly toss some protein into your daily diet. One of the coolest things about being vegan is taking really beneficial foods like lentils and recreating healthier versions of foods from the Standard American Diet that aren't so harsh on the digestive system. In this chapter you will see just how versatile lentils can be by way of falafel, tacos, sliders, stews, dips, and soups.

So whatever you might have thought about lentils before, erase it from your mind. Dive into a world of possibilities and discover just how easy and shockingly delicious lentils can be.

# THE BASICS OF COOKING LENTILS

You can cook lentils in advance and have them on hand to toss in meals for texture, flavor, and protein. I'm including a basic method to cook brown lentils, commonly labeled simply as "lentils" on the bag or in the bulk foods section of your market. Typically, red, green, and yellow lentils are labeled by color. They all cook up differently, have a different finish in terms of texture, and take different amounts of time to soften, so be sure to read the directions on the package if you go for something other than basic brown.

**1 cup dried brown lentils, rinsed and drained**
**3 cups water or low-sodium vegetable broth**

**1.** Combine the lentils and water in a medium pot and bring to a boil over medium–high heat. Cover and reduce the heat to a simmer.

**2.** Simmer for 15 to 20 minutes, until tender. Brown lentils will not be mushy when cooked properly; they will hold their shape.

**TIP:** *Cook lentils in vegetable broth to add more flavor to savory dishes.*

# Lentil-Walnut Dip

**GF** **30**

1 tablespoon olive oil

1 onion, chopped

1 (15-ounce) can lentils, rinsed
and drained

½ cup chopped walnuts

½ cup Mayonnaise (page 223) or
store-bought vegan mayonnaise

¼ teaspoon sea salt

**SERVES 8 TO 10 • PREP TIME: 5 MINUTES •
COOK TIME: 5 MINUTES**

This is a delicious dip that can be served with crackers
and veggies for an anytime snack or party dish. I urge
you to make it and then move directly on to the first
variation, the Thanksgiving Sandwich. This is one of my
favorite sandwiches in the world, and it is a home run
thanks to this very simple dip recipe.

**1.** Heat the oil in a medium skillet over medium heat.
Add the onion and sauté for 3 minutes, or until soft.

**2.** Transfer the onion to a blender and add the lentils,
walnuts, mayonnaise, and salt. Blend until smooth,
stopping periodically to scrape down the sides of the
blender with a spatula to ensure that all ingredients are
incorporated.

**3.** Transfer the mixture to a serving dish.

**VARIATIONS**

**THANKSGIVING SANDWICH:** Stack a vegan hoagie bun with
arugula, sliced apples, dried cranberries, and vegan
turkey deli slices. Slather with this dip for a handheld
Thanksgiving.

**SUN-DRIED TOMATO AND DILL LENTIL SPREAD:** Replace the
walnuts with 10 sun-dried tomatoes, chopped, and
2 teaspoons chopped fresh dill. Blend until smooth.

**TIP:** *The recipes in this book are designed for a standard
blender, but you still have to stop and occasionally scrape
down the sides. If you have a food processor, it will be
perfect for this recipe, but any blender will do the trick.*

# Warm Lentil Salad

**GF** **NF** **SF** 30

2 tablespoons olive oil, divided

1 onion, chopped

2 garlic cloves, minced

1 red bell pepper, seeded and diced

2 celery stalks, thinly sliced

1 teaspoon dried thyme

1 (15-ounce) can lentils, rinsed
and drained

1 tablespoon red wine vinegar

¼ teaspoon sea salt

¼ teaspoon black pepper

1 (5-ounce) package mixed
spring greens

**SERVES 4 • PREP TIME: 5 MINUTES • COOK TIME: 15 MINUTES**

My world changed when I discovered I could get cooked lentils in a can. Though they are easy to make out of the bag, it is great to be able to toss already-cooked lentils with other ingredients for a quick protein-packed snack or salad topper.

**1.** Heat 1 tablespoon of olive oil in a medium skillet over medium heat. Add the onion and sauté for 3 minutes, or until soft. Add the garlic and sauté for 1 additional minute, or until fragrant.

**2.** Add the remaining 1 tablespoon of oil to the skillet, along with the bell pepper, celery, and thyme. Mix well. Cook for 3 to 5 minutes, until the bell pepper is tender.

**3.** Add the lentils and vinegar. Stir well to combine, then add the salt and pepper. Taste and add more salt and pepper if desired. Cook for 2 more minutes, or until heated through.

**4.** Divide the mixed spring greens among 4 bowls and top with the lentil mixture.

### VARIATIONS

**ROASTED BABY POTATO AND WARM LENTIL SALAD:** Toss 1½ pounds halved baby potatoes with 1 tablespoon olive oil, ½ teaspoon salt, and ½ teaspoon black pepper. Spread out on a parchment-lined baking sheet and roast at 400°F for 30 minutes, flipping once with a spatula halfway through. Mix with the warm lentil salad, and serve atop the mixed spring greens.

**BALSAMIC CAPRESE LENTIL SALAD:** Replace the red wine vinegar with 1 to 2 tablespoons balsamic vinegar. Add 1 cup halved cherry tomatoes and 1 batch Fast Feta (page 225) and toss well to combine.

**TIP:** *The best way to deal with the problem of sodium in canned beans or lentils is to rinse them under running water. This will remove up to 60 percent of the sodium content.*

# One-Pot Dhal

**GF** **NF** **SF** **30**

1 (1-pound) bag dried red lentils

1 red bell pepper, seeded and diced

1 onion, chopped

3 garlic cloves, minced

1 teaspoon minced fresh ginger

5 cups low-sodium vegetable broth

Juice of ½ lemon

1 tablespoon curry powder

1 teaspoon sea salt

¼ teaspoon cayenne pepper
   (optional)

SERVES 4 TO 6 • PREP TIME: 10 MINUTES •
COOK TIME: 20 MINUTES

What I love most about dhal is that it is a comforting dish all year round. The sharp spices work just as well for me on a breezy summer evening as on a cold winter's night. In an effort to give you a quick and easy option, I call for curry powder instead of several individual spices. But if you like this dhal, delve deeper into the land of Indian spices to enlighten your senses one spice at a time.

**1.** In a large pot, combine the lentils, bell pepper, onion, garlic, ginger, broth, lemon juice, curry powder, salt and cayenne (if using).

**2.** Cover and bring to a boil over medium-high heat. Reduce the heat and simmer for 15 to 20 minutes, until the dhal has thickened and the lentils are soft.

### VARIATIONS

**TROPICAL DHAL:** Add cubed mango to your dhal after it has cooked.

**MOROCCAN DHAL:** Add ½ cup raisins and 2 cups baby spinach to the dhal after cooking. Stir well until the spinach is wilted.

**TIP:** *I prefer dhal to be very creamy. If you find you like yours that way as well, try simmering this dish for 5 to 10 more minutes, stirring frequently, until you reach the desired creaminess.*

# Spiced Lentil Tacos

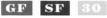

2 (15-ounce) cans lentils, rinsed and drained

1½ cups chunky mild salsa

1 tablespoon Taco Seasoning (page 219) or store-bought taco seasoning

12 taco shells

1½ cups shredded romaine lettuce

2 tomatoes, seeded and chopped

Sour Cream (page 222) or store-bought vegan sour cream

1 cup shredded carrot or vegan cheddar shreds

6 scallions, thinly sliced

**SERVES 6 · PREP TIME: 5 MINUTES · COOK TIME: 10 MINUTES**

Ways to my heart: Buy me tacos, make me tacos, *be* tacos. As Ariel sang in *The Little Mermaid*, "I want to be where the tacos are"—right? Okay, maybe she didn't say that exactly but I'm pretty sure that is what she meant. Who doesn't want to be where the tacos are?

**1.** In a large skillet, combine the lentils, salsa, and taco seasoning, and bring to a boil over medium-high heat. Reduce to a simmer and cook for 5 to 8 minutes, until the liquid reduces by half.

**2.** Build each taco by placing in the shell a layer of the lentil mixture, some lettuce, then tomatoes and sour cream. Top with the carrots and sprinkle with the scallions.

### VARIATIONS

**GREEK TACOS:** Omit the romaine lettuce, sour cream, and carrots. Instead, add baby spinach, sliced olives, and Fast Feta (page 225).

**SWEET POTATO AND LENTIL TACOS:** Use just 1 can of lentils. Peel 1 large sweet potato and cut into ½-inch pieces. Toss the potatoes with 1 teaspoon olive oil and spread out on a parchment-lined baking sheet. Roast at 400°F for 20 minutes, or until just fork-tender. Add the potatoes with the 1 can of lentils and continue with the recipe as written.

**TIP:** *Hard taco shells from the grocery store can seem somewhat stale, even fresh from the package. Warm them in the oven at 350°F for 5 minutes for a crispy shell.*

# Slow-Cooker Lentil and Vegetable Stew

**GF** **NF** **SF**

3 carrots, peeled and cut into
½-inch pieces

2 medium russet potatoes, cut into
1-inch pieces

2 celery stalks, thinly sliced

1 onion, chopped

4 garlic cloves, minced

1 (1-pound) bag dried lentils

6 cups low-sodium vegetable broth

1 bay leaf

2 teaspoons Italian seasoning

1 teaspoon sea salt

1 (5-ounce) package baby spinach

SERVES 10 TO 12 • PREP TIME: 15 MINUTES •
COOK TIME: 8 HOURS

I grew up in two houses; my parents were divorced and I would stay at my dad's on the weekends. My father wasn't exactly a culinary master, but he was all about us cooking together. I spent many weekends making biscuits from Jiffy mixes and warming up cans of Dinty Moore beef stew. While it wasn't so good for my health, I certainly have fond memories of cooking on those weekends. Any hearty stew reminds me of that, including this one.

**1.** In a slow cooker, combine the carrots, potatoes, celery, onion, garlic, lentils, broth, bay leaf, Italian seasoning, and salt. Mix well to combine. Cover and cook on low for 8 hours.

**2.** Remove the bay leaf. Mix the spinach into the stew and stir until wilted.

## VARIATIONS

**CHICKEN AND LENTIL STEW:** After 8 hours, add vegan chicken strips to the stew, cover, and cook on low for an additional 30 minutes. Then remove the bay leaf and stir in the spinach until wilted.

**LENTIL STEW AND DUMPLINGS:** In a medium bowl, lightly mix together 1 cup all-purpose flour, 1 tablespoon baking powder, ¼ teaspoon salt, and ¾ cup unsweetened soy or almond milk to make a dough. After 8 hours, remove the bay leaf and stir the spinach into the stew until wilted. Then drop the dumpling dough on top of the stew by heaping tablespoons. Cover and cook on high for an additional 30 minutes, or until the dumplings have increased in size and the dough has become dry.

**TIP:** *As mentioned in the opening of this chapter, brown lentils are labeled simply "lentils" in the store because they are the most common variety of lentil. They also have a firmer texture than most other lentils when cooked, making them perfect for a slow-cooker recipe.*

**NO SLOW COOKER? NO PROBLEM:** *To prepare this recipe on the stove, heat 1 tablespoon olive oil in a stockpot over medium heat. Add the onion and garlic and sauté for 2 minutes, or until fragrant. Add the remaining ingredients except the spinach, cover, and simmer for 50 to 60 minutes. Remove the bay leaf and add the spinach, stirring until wilted.*

# ntil Falafel

 30

Nonstick cooking spray

1 (15-ounce) can lentils, rinsed and drained

¼ cup flax meal

3 garlic cloves, minced

½ cup chopped fresh parsley

Juice of ½ lemon

1¼ teaspoons ground cumin

½ teaspoon sea salt

½ teaspoon black pepper

**SERVES 4 · PREP TIME: 10 MINUTES · COOK TIME: 20 MINUTES**

Falafel is traditionally made with chickpeas, but I have used all sorts of beans for this recipe. Now it's time for a lentil version. After all the variations I have made over the years, I always come back to this one, and it remains my favorite. I hope you enjoy it, too.

**1.** Preheat the oven to 425°F. Line a baking sheet with parchment paper and spray with nonstick cooking spray.

**2.** In a large bowl, combine all the ingredients. Mix well to combine and mash the mixture against the sides of the bowl with your spoon to create a doughy texture.

**3.** Form each falafel ball using 1 heaping tablespoon of dough. Place the balls on the prepared baking sheet and slightly flatten each ball into a disk. Spray the tops with nonstick cooking spray.

**4.** Bake for 10 minutes, flip, and bake for 10 more minutes, or until crispy.

### VARIATIONS

**FALAFEL PITA:** Stuff a whole-wheat pita with shredded romaine, chopped olives, chopped tomato, falafel, and hummus. Drizzle with sriracha, if desired.

**FALAFEL SALAD:** Create a bowl with spinach, Quinoa and Broccoli Tabbouleh (page 100), falafel, chopped tomatoes, and chopped olives. Add Fast Feta (page 225) for a robust flavor profile.

**TIP:** *If you prefer the traditional falafel made with chickpeas, use 1 (15-ounce) can chickpeas, rinsed, drained, and mashed.*

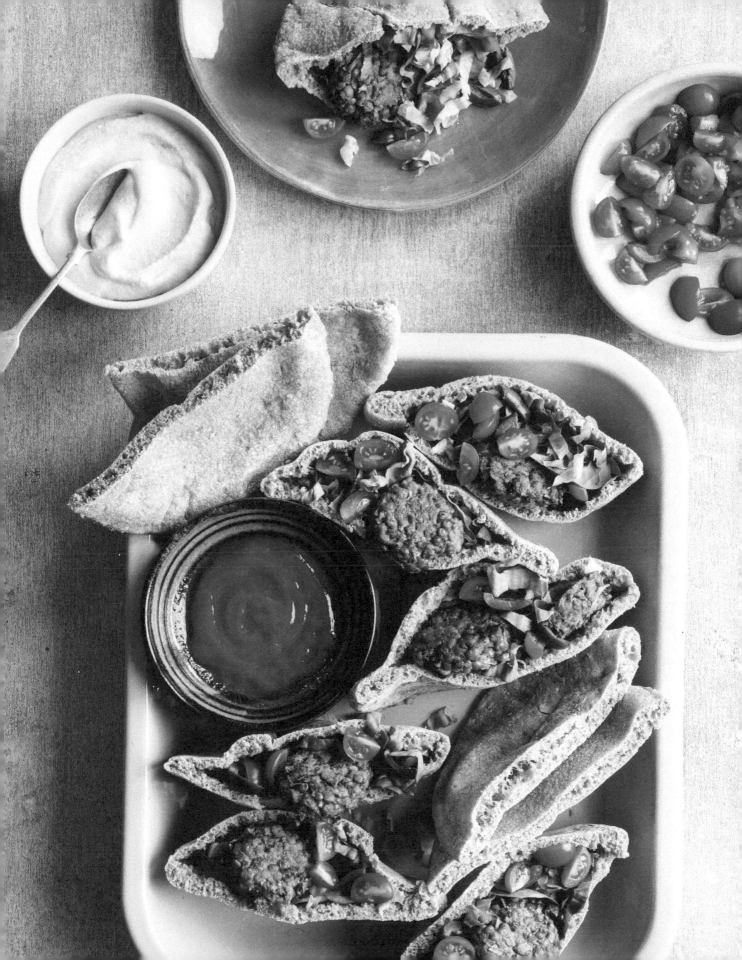

# Lentil Sliders

Nonstick cooking spray

2 teaspoons olive oil

½ cup chopped onion

3 garlic cloves, minced

1 (15-ounce) can lentils, rinsed
and drained

1 tablespoon soy sauce or
gluten-free tamari

½ cup vegan breadcrumbs

2 teaspoons Italian seasoning

8 vegan slider buns

Mustard, for serving

Ketchup, for serving

Pickle slices, for serving

**TIP:** *If you have trouble finding vegan slider buns, check out vegan dinner-roll options in your supermarket; they are usually the appropriate size. Just read the label to make sure they are vegan.*

**SERVES 4 TO 8 • PREP TIME: 10 MINUTES • COOK TIME: 25 MINUTES**

Sliders are always fun to serve at a party. I like to make a variety of them and stick little flags in them that suit the occasion. If you are having passed appetizers, these are a great addition because your guests can grab one and devour it in just a couple of bites without a plate or cutlery, leaving their other hand free for a cocktail!

**1.** Preheat the oven to 425°F. Line a baking sheet with parchment paper and spray with nonstick cooking spray.

**2.** Heat the oil in a large skillet over medium heat. Add the onion and sauté for 3 minutes, or until soft. Add the garlic and sauté for 1 additional minute, or until fragrant. Transfer the onion and garlic to a large bowl.

**3.** Add the lentils, soy sauce, breadcrumbs, and Italian seasoning to the bowl and mix until well combined. Use the back of your spoon to mash the mixture against the sides of the bowl, creating a dough-like texture.

**4.** Scoop out heaping ¼-cup portions of the lentil mixture and form each into a slider patty. Place the patties on the prepared baking sheet, and spray the tops with nonstick cooking spray. Bake for 10 minutes, flip, and bake for an additional 10 minutes, or until browned.

**5.** Transfer the sliders to buns and top with mustard, ketchup, and pickles.

### VARIATIONS

**ITALIAN MEATBALLS:** Instead of sliders, shape the dough into meatballs and bake as directed. Serve them with Magnificent Marinara (page 231) and pasta, topped with Walnut Parmesan (page 230) and chopped fresh basil.

**BBQ SLIDERS:** Omit the mustard, ketchup, and pickles. Top your sliders with Basic BBQ Sauce (page 232) and French's fried onions.

# Untidy Lentil Joes

 NF  30

1 tablespoon olive oil

1 onion, chopped

1 green bell pepper, seeded and chopped

2 garlic cloves, minced

2 (15-ounce) cans lentils, rinsed and drained

1 (15-ounce) can low-sodium tomato sauce

2 tablespoons vegan steak sauce

2 tablespoons dark-brown sugar

1 tablespoon chili powder

2 teaspoons ground cumin

8 whole-wheat vegan hamburger buns, toasted (see Tip)

**SERVES 8 • PREP TIME: 10 MINUTES • COOK TIME: 15 MINUTES**

The word *untidy* is a bit more refined than *sloppy*, but we're not fooling anyone; these are a delicious take on the sloppy Joe. I use A.1. steak sauce—yes, it's vegan! You'll want to triple or quadruple this recipe for backyard barbecues, parties, and family vacations.

**1.** Heat the oil in a large skillet over medium-high heat. Add the onion and bell pepper and sauté for 3 minutes. Lower the heat to medium, add the garlic, and sauté for 1 additional minute, or until fragrant. Add the lentils, mix well, and cook for 2 more minutes.

**2.** Add the tomato sauce, steak sauce, sugar, chili powder, and cumin. Mix well, cover, and simmer for 10 minutes. Season with salt and pepper, to taste.

**3.** Serve on toasted buns.

### VARIATIONS

**HEARTY UNTIDY LENTIL JOES:** Use just 1 can of lentils. Steam 1 (8-ounce) package tempeh for 15 minutes, then crumble it into the skillet along with the 1 can of lentils.

**UNTIDY KALE AND SWEET POTATO HASH:** Serve this over Kale and Sweet Potato Hash (page 33) for a complete meal.

**TIP:** *To get a tasty toast on your buns, spread vegan butter on each cut side and toast in a skillet over medium-high heat until the edges start to brown, about 2 minutes.*

# Lentil Bolognese

   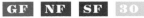

**GF** **NF** **SF** **30**

1 tablespoon olive oil

1 onion, chopped

2 carrots, peeled and grated

4 garlic cloves, minced

1 (15-ounce) can lentils, rinsed
and drained

1 tablespoon dark-brown sugar

2 teaspoons Italian seasoning

¼ teaspoon sea salt

Pinch red pepper flakes

1 recipe Magnificent Marinara
(page 231) or 3 cups store-bought
marinara

Cooked pasta, greens, or grains,
for serving

**SERVES 4 TO 6 • PREP TIME: 10 MINUTES •
COOK TIME: 15 MINUTES**

Spaghetti and sauce! There is literally nothing better. This is a perfect way to add some extra protein or even get the kids eating some nutrient-dense foods with their pasta. A little trickery is okay when it comes to getting anyone to eat healthier.

**1.** Heat the oil in a large skillet over medium heat. Add the onion and carrots and sauté for 5 minutes, or until the vegetables are soft. Add the garlic and sauté for 1 additional minute, or until fragrant.

**2.** Add the lentils, sugar, Italian seasoning, salt, and red pepper flakes and stir well to combine.

**3.** Add the marinara and simmer for 5 minutes, or until heated through. Serve hot on top of your favorite pasta, greens, or grains.

### VARIATIONS

**MEDITERRANEAN BOLOGNESE:** Replace the carrots with ½ cup chopped black olives and ½ cup quartered canned (rinsed and drained) artichokes.

**TEMPEH BOLOGNESE:** Omit the lentils. Steam 1 (8-ounce) package tempeh for 15 minutes, then crumble it into the skillet in place of the lentils.

**TIP:** *Bolognese is one of those sauces that come to life over time. While you can make this recipe quickly and serve it right away, consider letting it sit in the fridge overnight. The next day, reheat it in a sauce pot over low heat. Let it simmer for 4 to 6 minutes, until heated through.*

# Skillet Shepherd's Pie

**GF** **NF**

1 cup low-sodium vegetable broth

1 tablespoon cornstarch

2 teaspoons olive oil

½ cup chopped onion

2 garlic cloves, minced

1 (15-ounce) can lentils, rinsed and drained

1 (10-ounce) bag frozen vegetable medley of your choice

1½ teaspoons dried thyme

½ teaspoon sea salt

½ teaspoon black pepper

2½ cups Classic Mashed Potatoes (page 129)

**TIP:** *You absolutely do not need a cast iron skillet to make all your shepherd's pie dreams a reality. Use a standard pie pan, any oven-safe skillet, or even an 8-inch baking dish. They are not as big as the skillet; they will be off by an inch or so. Be sure to adjust the amount of filling accordingly, as it will bubble up and out if you put in too much. You might want to place a baking sheet on the rack below the baking dish in the oven to catch any overflow.*

SERVES 8 · PREP TIME: 10 MINUTES · COOK TIME: 30 MINUTES

Shepherd's pie is commonly known as a cottage or meat pie, with a topping of mashed potatoes instead of pie crust. While my version was not created in a cottage and does not have meat, I can guarantee it satisfies anyone who falls in the "meat and potatoes" category, like myself—which is exactly why I created a tremendously easy vegan version of this classic.

**1.** Preheat the oven to 425°F.

**2.** In a small bowl, whisk together the broth and cornstarch to create a slurry, and set aside.

**3.** In a 10-inch cast iron skillet, heat the oil over medium heat. Add the onion and sauté for 3 minutes, or until soft. Add the garlic and sauté for 1 additional minute, or until fragrant.

**4.** Add the lentils, frozen vegetables, thyme, salt, and pepper, mix well, and sauté for 2 minutes, or until heated through.

**5.** Slowly stir in the cornstarch slurry. Cook for 3 to 5 minutes, until the mixture thickens. Remove from the heat.

**6.** Spread a layer of mashed potatoes on top of everything in the skillet. (If the potatoes are too thick, add a little water or nondairy milk to the mash before layering it on top.) Bake for 18 to 20 minutes, until bubbling.

## VARIATIONS

**SWEET POTATO SHEPHERD'S PIE:** Make Classic Mashed Potatoes (page 129) using the sweet potato variation.

**ETHIOPIAN SHEPHERD'S PIE:** Instead of the lentils, use the recipe for Ethiopian Cabbage, Carrot, and Potato Stew (page 36). Top with classic or sweet mashed potatoes.

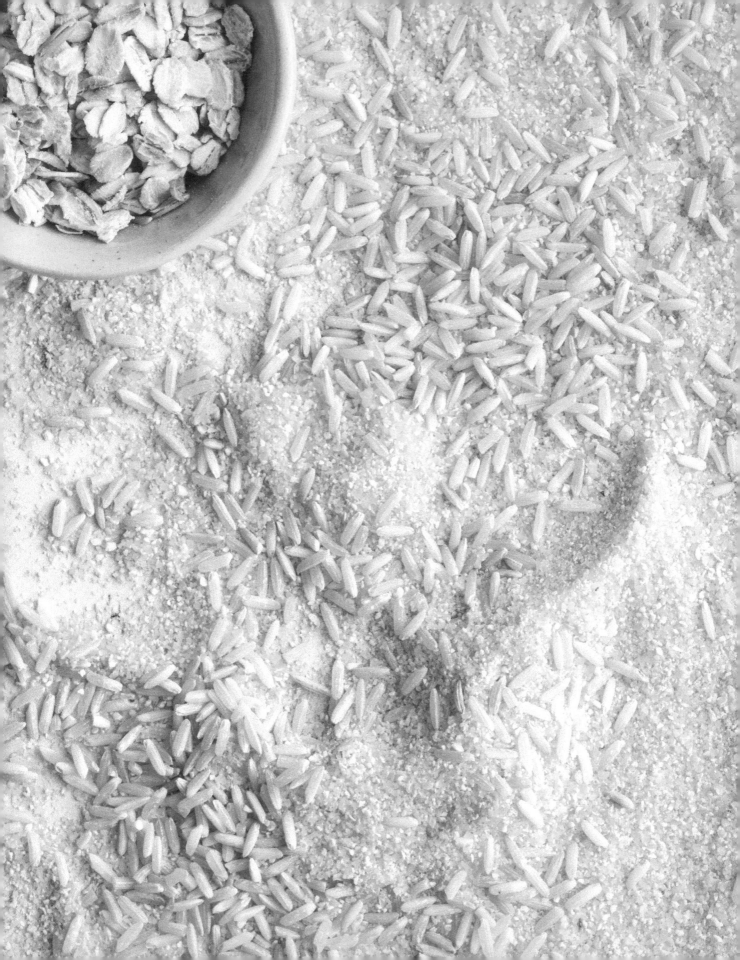

# CHAPTER 5

# Grains

Research tells us that whole grains are good for us. Hooray! But don't go crazy diving into whole-wheat pretzels, organic corn chips, or "enriched" Wonder Bread slices. Stick with making your grains from scratch whenever you can, and avoid the packaged and processed.

Grains have been cultivated and part of the human diet for thousands of years, which is another perfectly sensible reason to eat them whole, unprocessed, and cooked from scratch, as nature intended.

If you are now saying to yourself, "Absolutely not! I want my instant brown rice," you do you, friend; get your grains in any way that works best for you! I support you. But I'm including some basic cooking methods for each grain included in this section, for that moment when you decide you are ready to make your first pot of rice, oats, quinoa, or polenta.

# THE BASICS OF COOKING GRAINS

Most recipes that use grains in this book call for the grain to be already cooked. Feel free to follow these basic cooking methods, or the instructions that come on the bag or box of grain you bought. If you are a price chopper, I know you shopped in the bulk section, so these basic methods are for you!

## BROWN RICE

1 cup medium-grain brown rice

2½ cups water

1 tablespoon olive oil (optional)

¼ teaspoon sea salt

**1.** Combine the rice, water, oil (if using), and salt in a medium saucepot, cover, and bring to a boil over medium-high heat. Reduce the heat and simmer for 40 to 45 minutes, until the water is absorbed.

**2.** Remove from the heat and let sit, covered, for 10 minutes. Fluff with a fork. This makes about 1⅔ cups of cooked rice.

## OATS

2 cups water

¼ teaspoon sea salt

1 cup rolled oats

**1.** In a medium saucepot, bring the water and salt to a boil over medium-high heat. Add the rolled oats. Reduce the heat and simmer, stirring occasionally, for 10 to 12 minutes, until creamy.

**2.** Remove from the heat and let stand for 2 minutes to thicken slightly. (At this point you can add your favorite toppings and sweetener, if desired.) This makes about 2 cups of cooked oats.

## QUINOA

2 cups water

1 cup quinoa, rinsed and drained

**1.** Combine the water and quinoa in a medium saucepot, cover, and bring to a boil over medium-high heat. Reduce the heat and simmer for 12 to 15 minutes, until all the liquid is absorbed.

**2.** Remove from the heat and let sit, covered, for 10 minutes. Fluff with a fork. This makes about 3 cups of cooked quinoa.

**TIP:** *Rinsing the quinoa removes its natural coating, saponin, which can make it taste bitter or soapy. Boxed quinoa is often pre-rinsed, but it never hurts to give it another rinse before using it.*

## POLENTA

6 cups water

½ teaspoon sea salt

2 cups polenta or yellow cornmeal

3 tablespoons vegan butter (optional)

**1.** In a large stockpot, bring the water and salt to a boil over medium-high heat. Gradually add the polenta in a steady stream, whisking continuously. Once the polenta has been completely whisked in, continue stirring frequently with a spoon to prevent sticking. Use a long-handle spoon to keep your hands safe, because the mixture will pop and bubble as you are stirring. It will take about 30 minutes until the mixture is very thick.

**2.** Stir in the vegan butter, if you wish. (You can also add seasoning if desired, such as more salt, black pepper, dried oregano, dried basil, or Italian seasoning blend.)

**3.** Serve creamy, or transfer to a mold and let sit for 10 minutes. Pop out of the mold and serve immediately; it will hold its shape. This makes about 6 cups of cooked polenta.

**TIP:** *For a sheet of prepared polenta that you can use for recipes in this chapter in place of a "prepared polenta tube," transfer the cooked mixture to a parchment-lined baking sheet and spread it out to the size of the sheet, creating a ¼- to ½-inch-thick layer of polenta. Place in the refrigerator to set for 2 to 3 hours or overnight. Cut into the desired shape and sear, grill, or bake. If you're using this in place of a prepared polenta tube, use a 2½-inch cookie cutter or open rim of a drinking glass to get the round shape.*

# Banana Cream Pie Smoothie

 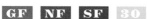  
**GF** **NF** **SF** 30

1 banana, frozen

1 cup unsweetened soy or almond milk

¼ cup uncooked rolled oats

1 tablespoon maple syrup

Pinch ground cinnamon

Pinch sea salt

SERVES 1 · PREP TIME: 5 MINUTES

I don't put greens in *all* my smoothies; sometimes I make them because I want something that tastes truly sinful. This decadent and creamy smoothie satisfies my sweet tooth every time. While this isn't a green smoothie, it's certainly a heck of a lot better for me than a slice of pie or a doughnut, and I still feel like I'm treating myself!

Combine all the ingredients in a blender and blend until smooth. Serve immediately.

### VARIATIONS

**BOSTON CREAM PIE:** Add 1 tablespoon fair-trade unsweetened cocoa powder.

**VELVET PEANUT BUTTER CHOCOLATE PIE:** Add 1 tablespoon fair-trade unsweetened cocoa powder and 2 tablespoons creamy peanut butter.

**TIP:** *Oats have a slight natural sweetness; if you are cutting back on calories, this recipe is still delicious without the maple syrup.*

# Peanut Butter Cup Overnight Oats

½ cup uncooked rolled oats

½ cup unsweetened soy or
almond milk

2 tablespoons natural creamy
peanut butter

2 tablespoons vegan chocolate chips

2 teaspoons sweetener of your choice

SERVES 1 · PREP TIME: 5 MINUTES, PLUS OVERNIGHT IN THE
REFRIGERATOR

I created this little mason jar of bliss when I first went vegan and was struggling to feel satisfied with my meals when I traveled. I would get particularly frustrated by the continental breakfasts at hotels, watching people dig into decadent pancakes and waffles, knowing very well how easily they could be made vegan. So I came up with this creation during the overnight-oats craze, and it has served me well. Pop it in the refrigerator before you go to bed, and you have oatmeal in the morning.

**1.** Mix all the ingredients in an 8-ounce container, cover, and refrigerate overnight.

**2.** In the morning, stir and enjoy.

### VARIATIONS

**TRAIL-MIX OVERNIGHT OATS:** Omit the peanut butter. Use only 1 tablespoon chocolate chips, plus 1 tablespoon dried fruit of your choice (chopped up, if the pieces are large), 1 tablespoon raw nuts of your choice, and 2 teaspoons maple syrup along with the oats and milk.

**MOCHA CRUNCH CHOCOLATE OVERNIGHT OATS:** Replace the peanut butter with 1½ teaspoons fair-trade unsweetened cocoa powder and ½ teaspoon instant espresso powder.

**TIP:** *I mix up a plastic container of this without the milk before I travel (you can put it in your carry-on as long as there isn't any liquid in it). When I get to my destination, I just get a small container of nondairy milk for my hotel fridge and mix it up. I've been known to pack a variety of these mixes and make my vacation companions very jealous!*

# Cinnamon Toast Crunch Granola

 **GF** 30

3 cups uncooked rolled oats

½ cup vegan butter, melted

¼ cup chopped raw almonds

¼ cup maple syrup

¼ cup plus 2 tablespoons organic cane sugar, divided

3 teaspoons ground cinnamon, divided

½ teaspoon vanilla extract

½ teaspoon sea salt

**SERVES 6 · PREP TIME: 5 MINUTES · COOK TIME: 15 MINUTES**

Who hasn't had a love affair with Cinnamon Toast Crunch cereal? I know I have, and I know I loved every second of it. I enjoy making it in granola form, too, because now I'm aware of all the ingredients that are in it. If you look at a box of cereal, you will see a lot of fillers and ingredients that are hard to pronounce, which is exactly why I put this classic cereal together instead.

**1.** Preheat the oven to 375°F. Line a baking sheet with parchment paper.

**2.** In a large bowl, mix together the oats, butter, almonds, maple syrup, ¼ cup cane sugar, 2 teaspoons cinnamon, vanilla, and salt.

**3.** Spread the mixture in a single layer on the prepared baking sheet. Bake for 10 minutes, toss with a spatula, and bake for an additional 5 minutes, or until lightly browned.

**4.** Remove from the oven and sprinkle with the remaining 2 tablespoons of cane sugar and 1 teaspoon of cinnamon.

**5.** Cool, and enjoy as a topping on a smoothie bowl or as a cereal combined with nondairy milk.

**VARIATIONS**

**CHAI-SPICED GRANOLA:** Omit the sugar and almonds, and take the oats down to 2 cups. Add 1 ½ cups crushed pecans, ½ teaspoon almond extract, 1 teaspoon ground cardamom, 1 teaspoon ground ginger, ¼ teaspoon ground allspice, and ¼ teaspoon ground cloves. Mix it all together, including the vanilla and salt, and bake as indicated.

**CINNAMON TRAIL-MIX GRANOLA:** Omit the almonds, and take the oats down to 2 cups. Add 1 cup raw nuts of your choice to the other ingredients and bake as directed. Mix in ½ cup dried fruit after the granola has cooled.

**TIP:** *Stored in a sealed container, granola can keep for up to 3 weeks in the pantry.*

# Savory Rosemary–Parmesan Granola

2 cups uncooked rolled oats

1 cup roughly chopped pecans

1 cup roughly chopped raw almonds

6 tablespoons olive oil

¼ cup Walnut Parmesan (page 230), nutritional yeast, or store-bought vegan Parmesan

2 teaspoons dried rosemary

1 teaspoon garlic powder

½ teaspoon sea salt

½ teaspoon black pepper

**SERVES 8 · PREP TIME: 5 MINUTES · COOK TIME: 20 MINUTES**

Granola isn't just for your sweet tooth! Savory recipes like this are great on salads, as a snack, sprinkled inside your favorite sandwich, or on top of rice dishes like Peas and Pesto Rice (page 94) or Coconut-Ginger Rice with Edamame (page 95). This granola can be stored in an airtight container for up to 3 weeks.

**1.** Preheat the oven to 375°F. Line a baking sheet with parchment paper.

**2.** In a large bowl, combine all the ingredients. Spread the mixture in an even layer on the prepared baking sheet. Bake for 10 minutes, toss with a spatula, and bake for an additional 5 minutes, or until lightly browned.

### VARIATIONS

**SAVORY THAI GRANOLA:** Combine 2 cups uncooked rolled oats, 1 cup pumpkin seeds, 3 tablespoons soy sauce or gluten-free tamari, 2 tablespoons olive oil, 1 tablespoon maple syrup, 1 teaspoon garlic powder, and ¼ teaspoon red pepper flakes. Bake as directed.

**SAVORY CURRY GRANOLA:** Combine 2 cups uncooked rolled oats, 1 cup chopped walnuts, ¼ cup olive oil, 1 tablespoon curry powder, and ½ teaspoon salt. Bake as directed, then add ½ cup raisins after it has cooled.

**TIP:** *Let's settle this once and for all: You can absolutely have oats if you are gluten-free! Oats are naturally gluten-free. The problem is in their processing. Be careful to purchase oats that are not only labeled gluten-free but are also certified gluten-free with an official GFCO (Gluten-Free Certification Organization) label, which means they have not been packaged in a factory with foods that contain gluten.*

# Blueberry Oatmeal Breakfast Bars

NF

2 cups uncooked rolled oats

2 cups all-purpose flour

1½ cups dark-brown sugar

1½ teaspoons baking soda

½ teaspoon sea salt

½ teaspoon ground cinnamon

1 cup vegan butter, melted

4 cups blueberries, fresh or frozen

¼ cup organic cane sugar

2 tablespoons cornstarch

MAKES 12 • PREP TIME: 10 MINUTES • COOK TIME: 40 MINUTES

These breakfast bars are great to have on hand for a quick breakfast or snack—or even a dessert, as they are on the sweeter side. I once took these to a picnic with a bunch of friends in Central Park, and they were a delightful addition to the standard offerings of pasta salad and sandwiches. They were the first thing at the picnic to disappear!

1. Preheat the oven to 375°F. Lightly grease a 9-by-13-inch baking dish.

2. In a large bowl, combine the oats, flour, sugar, baking soda, salt, and cinnamon. Add the butter and mix until well incorporated and crumbly.

3. In a separate large bowl, combine the blueberries, cane sugar, and cornstarch, mixing until the blueberries are evenly coated.

4. Press 3 cups of the oatmeal mixture into the prepared baking pan. Spread the blueberry mixture on top and crumble the remaining oatmeal mixture over the blueberries. Bake for 40 minutes.

5. Remove from the oven and let cool completely before cutting into bars.

## VARIATIONS

**MIXED BERRY BREAKFAST BARS:** Take it down to 1 cup blueberries, and add 1 cup sliced strawberries, 1 cup raspberries, and 1 cup blackberries.

**RASPBERRY LEMONADE BREAKFAST BARS:** Omit the blueberries. Add 4 cups fresh or frozen raspberries and 1 tablespoon lemon extract.

TIP: *Cornstarch is a thickener. Make sure it coats all the fruit evenly in this mixture so the recipe thickens throughout.*

# Warm Quinoa Breakfast Bowl

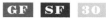

3 cups freshly cooked quinoa

1⅓ cups unsweetened soy or almond milk

2 bananas, sliced

1 cup raspberries

1 cup blueberries

½ cup chopped raw walnuts

¼ cup maple syrup

**SERVES 4 • PREP TIME: 5 MINUTES**

I featured a bowl like this in the Boston episode of *The Vegan Roadie.* Loaded with protein, bright fruits, and savory nuts, this dish has all the textures and flavors I want to start my day off right. I hope it finds a spot in your breakfast lineup.

**1.** Divide the ingredients among 4 bowls, starting with a base of ¾ cup quinoa, ⅓ cup milk, ½ banana, ¼ cup raspberries, ¼ cup blueberries, and 2 tablespoons walnuts.

**2.** Drizzle 1 tablespoon of maple syrup over the top of each bowl.

**VARIATIONS**

**PROTEIN POWER BOWL:** Add chia and hemp seeds for a protein-packed breakfast.

**TROPICAL QUINOA BOWL:** Replace the raspberries and blueberries with diced mango and pineapple and top with some unsweetened shredded coconut.

**TIP:** *Make the quinoa ahead of time and warm it up in the microwave for a quick breakfast bowl.*

# Quinoa Nachos Supreme

GF 30

½ cup salsa

¼ cup uncooked quinoa

¼ cup water

1 teaspoon soy sauce or gluten-free tamari

½ teaspoon chili powder

Tortilla chips

¾ cup canned black beans, rinsed and drained

½ cup Easy Cheese Sauce–Nacho variation (page 224) or store-bought vegan cheddar shreds

½ cup seeded and chopped tomato

½ cup shredded purple cabbage

¼ cup Sour Cream (page 222) or store-bought vegan sour cream

2 scallions, chopped

SERVES 4 TO 6 · PREP TIME: 10 MINUTES · COOK TIME: 15 MINUTES

Nachos are everything! I have traveled this country far and wide and have had some of the best vegan nacho plates in all the land. Now that it's time for me to finally share a recipe of my own, I draw on inspiration from FüD in Kansas City, Missouri, and San Antonio restaurants Viva Vegeria and Señor Veggie. All fantastic places, if you ever find yourself in those parts . . . and if you do, definitely get the nachos! Until then, make them yourself.

**1.** In a medium saucepot, combine the salsa, quinoa, water, soy sauce, and chili powder. Cover and bring to a boil over medium-high heat. Reduce to a simmer and cook, covered, for 15 minutes, or until all the water is absorbed. Remove from the heat and let stand 5 minutes, then fluff with a fork.

**2.** On a large platter build your nachos starting with a layer of tortilla chips, then beans, quinoa, cheese sauce (see Tip if using store-bought cheese shreds), tomato, and cabbage. Add another layer of chips, beans, quinoa, cheese, tomato, and cabbage. Finish off the nachos by drizzling the sour cream over the top and sprinkling with the scallions.

### VARIATIONS

**MEATY NACHOS:** Omit the quinoa. Add ¾ cup vegan beef crumbles or vegan chicken strips seasoned with 1 to 2 tablespoons Taco Seasoning (page 219).

**HAWAIIAN NACHOS:** Replace the tomato with cubed mango or pineapple, and drizzle with Basic BBQ Sauce (page 232) instead of sour cream.

**TIP:** *If you're using store-bought vegan cheese shreds, layer everything except the sour cream and scallions on an oven-safe platter or baking dish. Bake at 425°F for 8 to 10 minutes to melt the cheese. Carefully set the platter on a second platter, drizzle with sour cream, and sprinkle with scallions. Warn your guest that the main platter is hot!*

# Rainbow Quinoa Salad

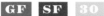 **GF** **SF** 30

SERVES 6 TO 8 • PREP TIME: 15 MINUTES

3 tablespoons olive oil

Juice of 1½ lemons

1 teaspoon garlic powder

½ teaspoon dried oregano

1 bunch curly kale, stemmed and roughly chopped

2 cups cooked tricolor quinoa

1 cup canned mandarin oranges in juice, drained

1 cup diced yellow summer squash

1 red bell pepper, seeded and diced

½ red onion, thinly sliced

½ cup dried cranberries or cherries

½ cup slivered almonds

Yes, vegans eat more than salad. This book, and all the ones that came before it, are obviously proof of that! Just the same, nobody does a salad quite like the vegans do, and it's not because it's the only thing to eat. It's because vegetables lightly dressed are refreshing, filling, and best of all, wonderful for us. So throw together this large bowl of nutritionally delicious goodness and share with family and friends, or eat it throughout the week.

**1.** In a small bowl, whisk together the oil, lemon juice, garlic powder, and oregano.

**2.** In a large bowl, toss the kale with the oil–lemon mixture until well coated. Add the quinoa, oranges, squash, bell pepper, and red onion and toss until all the ingredients are well combined.

**3.** Divide among bowls or transfer to a large serving platter. Top with the cranberries and almonds.

### VARIATIONS

**PROTEIN RAINBOW SALAD:** Add 1 cup chopped vegan chicken, Basic Baked Tofu (page 137), or another plant-based protein, along with ¼ cup chia seeds.

**CHOPPY CRUNCH RAINBOW SALAD:** Add some almond crunch from the Almond Crunch Chopped Kale Salad (page 16) and ¼ cup hemp seeds for a delightful crunchy salad. Lay it all out on a cutting board in a couple of batches and chop with a large chef's knife.

**TIP:** *The most effective way to taste-test dressing is to dip one leaf into the dressing and adjust the seasoning, if desired, before adding the dressing to all the greens.*

# Quinoa Collard Wraps

 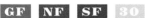

**GF** **NF** **SF** 30

4 large collard green leaves

¼ cup White Bean Hummus (page 43) or store-bought hummus

½ cup cooked quinoa

1 avocado, peeled, pitted, and sliced

½ cup julienned or grated carrot

½ cup shredded or thinly sliced purple cabbage

**SERVES 4 • PREP TIME: 10 MINUTES**

Finding ways to cut carbs has always been a struggle for me. I love my bread. But I also love the way I feel when I'm able to trim the carbs down. Wrapping your favorite sandwich ingredients in a sturdy green leaf is an excellent alternative, and it lets you keep things lean, green, and clean. Try this recipe as is, and then get crafty and personalize it with other ingredients you love.

**1.** Remove the thick bottom part of the stem from each collard leaf. Lay 1 leaf on a flat surface with the stem-side facing away from you.

**2.** Spread 1 tablespoon hummus down the center of the wrap, followed by 2 tablespoons quinoa, a few avocado slices, 2 tablespoons carrot, and 2 tablespoons cabbage.

**3.** Fold in the sides of the leaf first, then fold the larger part of the leaf, the part closest to you, over the filling. Start rolling up until everything is held snug inside.

**4.** Slice on a diagonal in the middle and secure with toothpicks, if necessary. Repeat with the remaining leaves and filling.

### VARIATIONS

**MEXI QUINOA AND PEACHES WRAP:** Replace the carrot and cabbage with sliced fresh peaches. Add hot sauce to taste.

**SOUTHWEST BURGER WRAP:** Omit the hummus, quinoa, carrot, and cabbage. Cut 2 Southwest Pinto Bean Burger (page 56) patties in half. Place a patty half horizontally on the leaf, along with some avocado slices and a spoonful of salsa, and roll up as directed.

**TIP:** *If you find your leaf is breaking when you roll it, double up the leaves to create a stronger wrap.*

# Peas and Pesto Rice

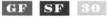
**GF** **SF** 30

1 cup Pistachio Pesto (page 226) or
 store-bought vegan pesto

1 cup frozen peas, thawed

2 cups cooked brown rice

**SERVES 2 TO 4 • PREP TIME: 5 MINUTES • COOK TIME: 5 MINUTES**

Pesto is one of those sauces that goes great on everything!
I was eating at a macrobiotic restaurant on the Lower
East Side in New York City and I had the most delicious
bowl that was simply pesto, tofu, kale, and brown rice. I
feel like this recipe is a nice base for all kinds of add-ons:
Add it to a salad or pair it with a protein if you want. Side
dish or main event, it's certain to satisfy.

**1.** In a large skillet, warm the pesto sauce and peas over low
heat for 3 to 5 minutes, until heated through.

**2.** Add the rice and mix until everything is coated.

## VARIATIONS

**PESTO PLATE:** Use 1 batch Basic Baked Tofu (page 137)
and 1 bunch curly kale, stemmed, roughly chopped, and
massaged in 1 teaspoon olive oil. Divide the Peas and
Pesto Rice, tofu, and kale among 4 plates for a mean green
machine of a dinner!

**VEGGIES AND PESTO RICE:** Warm 1 tablespoon olive oil in a
large skillet over medium heat and sauté ½ onion, chopped,
1 zucchini, diced, and 1 (8-ounce) package baby bella or
white button mushrooms, stemmed and sliced. Mix with the
rice and a double batch of Pistachio Pesto.

**TIP:** *Pesto oxidizes and turns brown when exposed to the air.
If you have leftovers of this dish (not likely!), you can avoid
this unsightly issue by covering your Peas and Pesto Rice
with a film of plastic wrap set directly on top of the rice.
Then refrigerate until you're ready to finish it off.*

# Coconut-Ginger Rice with Edamame

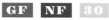 

SERVES 4 TO 6 · PREP TIME: 5 MINUTES · COOK TIME: 15 MINUTES

1 cup low-sodium vegetable broth

1 cup uncooked jasmine rice

½ cup full-fat coconut milk

2 teaspoons minced fresh ginger

¼ teaspoon sea salt

Juice of ½ lemon

¾ cup fresh or frozen (and thawed) shelled edamame

The recipe name suggests that every bite is going to be warm and comforting, and it is. If you love coconut, you can't go wrong cooking the rice in coconut milk, with a subtle spike of ginger and lemon to elevate it. Toss in some edamame for texture and protein, and that's one delicious dish! You can often find edamame in the frozen-food section with the vegetables, still in the pod or already shelled.

**1.** Combine the broth, rice, coconut milk, ginger, and salt in a medium saucepot. Give it a good stir to incorporate the ginger. Cover the pot and bring to a boil over medium-high heat. Reduce the heat and simmer for 15 minutes, or until all the liquid is absorbed and the rice is tender (see Tip).

**2.** Remove the pot from the heat and let sit for 5 minutes. Add the lemon juice and edamame and fluff with a fork.

### VARIATIONS

**COCONUT-CRANBERRY RICE:** Omit the lemon juice and edamame. Instead, at the end add 1 tablespoon orange juice and ¾ cup dried cranberries.

**COCONUT RICE SALAD:** Turn this simple side dish into a meal. After the rice is cooked, add ¾ cup dried cranberries or cherries, ½ cup chopped walnuts, 2 chopped scallions, 2 tablespoons orange juice, ¼ teaspoon salt, and ¼ teaspoon black pepper. Serve atop a bed of chopped romaine or curly kale.

**TIP:** *Don't lift the lid at all during the cooking time! Wait until the 15 minutes are up and then check the liquid absorption by inserting a butter knife into the center of the rice and moving the rice to the side to get a look at the bottom of the pan. You shouldn't see any liquid.*

# Stovetop Thanksgiving Rice Stuffing

**GF** **30**

¼ cup vegan butter

1 onion, chopped

2 celery stalks, thinly sliced

1 (8-ounce) package baby bella or white button mushrooms, stemmed and sliced

3 garlic cloves, minced

½ cup low-sodium vegetable broth

½ cup dried cranberries or cherries

½ cup chopped walnuts, toasted

2 cups cooked wild-rice blend or brown rice

1 teaspoon poultry seasoning

1 teaspoon sea salt

Chopped fresh parsley, for garnish

**SERVES 8 TO 10 • PREP TIME: 10 MINUTES • COOK TIME: 15 MINUTES**

Who doesn't love the stuffing at Thanksgiving? I never sacrifice that as a vegan, though it is weird to call it stuffing, right? Enter gluten-free guests who are also vegan—what to do? This recipe is the answer. If guests have a nut allergy, simply replace the walnuts with sunflower or pumpkin seeds to keep the same texture.

**1.** Melt the butter in a large skillet over medium heat. Add the onion, celery, and mushrooms and sauté for 5 minutes, or until soft. Add the garlic and sauté for 1 additional minute, or until fragrant.

**2.** Add the broth, cranberries, and walnuts. Bring to a boil, cover, reduce the heat, and simmer for 5 minutes, or until fragrant.

**3.** Add the rice, poultry seasoning, and salt and mix well to combine. Continue to cook, uncovered, for 4 minutes, stirring occasionally, or until heated through and all the liquid evaporates.

**4.** Transfer to a serving dish and garnish with parsley.

### VARIATIONS

**GLUTTONY STOVETOP RICE STUFFING:** Stir in 2 cups seasoned croutons just after you cook the rice for 4 minutes, and let sit for 2 minutes for the croutons to absorb the juices.

**SAUSAGE STUFFING:** Sear 4 vegan sausage links, sliced, in a separate pan in 1 tablespoon olive oil to crisp them up. Add the sausage when you add the rice.

**TIP:** *Make this item ahead of the holiday rush. You can cook it the day before and reheat it the day of the gathering in a large skillet over low heat. Stir in a couple tablespoons of water to add some moisture and keep it from sticking to the skillet.*

# Picture-Perfect Paella

GF NF SF 30

1 tablespoon olive oil

1 onion, chopped

1 red bell pepper, seeded and sliced

3 garlic cloves, minced

1 tomato, diced

1 cup frozen peas, thawed

1 cup canned artichokes, drained, rinsed, and quartered

1 tablespoon paprika

1 teaspoon ground turmeric

1½ teaspoons sea salt

2 cups cooked brown rice

Chopped fresh parsley, for garnish (optional)

SERVES 4 TO 6 • PREP TIME: 10 MINUTES • COOK TIME: 15 MINUTES

Paella is one of those dishes that are easily veganized. While this recipe calls for bell peppers, peas, and artichokes, you can add just about whatever you want to this dish. If you have a garden and want to toss in your favorite seasonal veggies, I encourage you to do so! Serve it up at the dinner table as your seasonal paella, and your guests will swoon.

**1.** Heat the oil in a large skillet over medium heat. Add the onion and bell pepper and sauté for 3 to 5 minutes, until soft. Add the garlic and sauté for 1 additional minute, or until fragrant.

**2.** Add the tomato, peas, artichokes, paprika, turmeric, and salt. Cook for 4 minutes, or until heated through.

**3.** Add the rice and mix well to combine. Serve hot, garnished with parsley, if desired.

### VARIATIONS

**SAUSAGE PAELLA:** For a heartier paella, omit the artichokes. Sauté 1 cup sliced vegan sausage with the onion and bell pepper.

**VALENCIAN-STYLE PAELLA:** Omit the bell pepper and peas. Add 1 cup trimmed fresh green beans and 1 cup canned white beans, rinsed and drained.

**TIP:** *To quickly thaw your peas, set them in a bowl in your sink and fill the bowl with hot water. The peas should thaw within minutes.*

# Veggie and Brown Rice Stir-Fry

**NF** **30**

**FOR THE SAUCE**

¾ cup low-sodium vegetable broth

2 tablespoons soy sauce or gluten-free tamari

1 tablespoon ketchup

1 tablespoon minced fresh ginger

3 garlic cloves, minced

2 teaspoons cornstarch

**FOR THE STIR-FRY**

1 tablespoon olive oil

1 red onion, cut into large chunks

3 cups bite-size broccoli florets

1 red bell pepper, seeded and diced

1 (8-ounce) package baby bella or white button mushrooms, stemmed and halved

4 cups cooked brown rice

SERVES 4 • PREP TIME: 10 MINUTES • COOK TIME: 10 MINUTES

Stir-fry is one of the most flexible meals you can make. Start with this recipe as your base in stir-fry land, but after that, what you toss in is up to you. Cook up your next stir-fry using this outline—maybe the same sauce but with the veggies of your choice. Or you can just stick with this one if you like it as much as I do. Be the kitchen warrior in your own home!

**1.** *To make the sauce:* In a small bowl, whisk together all the sauce ingredients.

**2.** *To make the stir-fry:* In a large skillet or wok, heat the oil over medium-high heat. Add the red onion, broccoli, bell pepper, and mushrooms and sauté for 6 to 8 minutes, until the vegetables reduce slightly in size and the broccoli is bright green.

**3.** Quickly give your sauce mixture another whisk, being sure to scrape up any settled cornstarch from the bottom of the bowl. Reduce the heat to medium and slowly stir the cornstarch mixture into the vegetables to avoid spattering. Cook for 2 minutes, or until thick, stirring occasionally.

**4.** Divide the rice among 4 bowls and top with the stir-fried veggies.

**VARIATIONS**

**CHICKEN OR BEEF STIR-FRY:** Replace the bell pepper and mushrooms with 2 cups vegan chicken or beef tips.

**QUINOA, TOFU, AND BROCCOLI STIR-FRY:** Replace the onion, bell pepper, and mushrooms with 1 batch Basic Baked Tofu (page 137). Replace the brown rice with 4 cups cooked quinoa.

**TIP:** *A large broccoli floret is going to take longer to cook than a tiny minced onion, so try to cut all your stir-fry vegetables to roughly the same size—bite-size works best. This will ensure even cooking.*

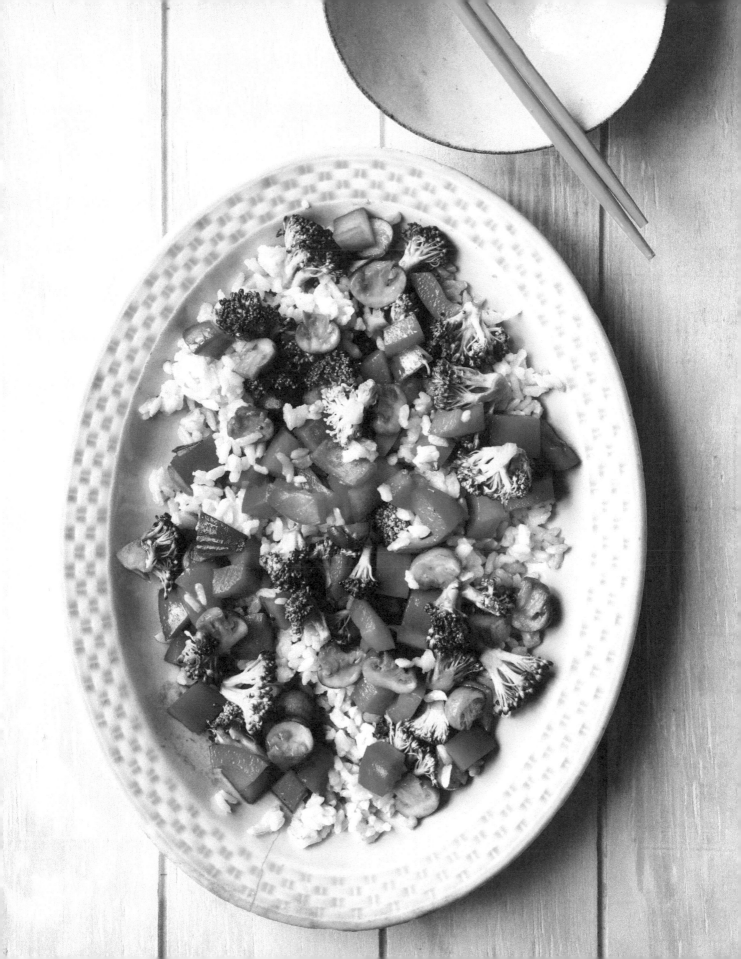

# Quinoa and Broccoli Tabbouleh

GF NF SF 30

1½ cups cooked quinoa

2 cups grated or finely chopped broccoli florets

1 cup peeled and diced cucumber

1 cup halved cherry tomatoes

2 tablespoons olive oil

Juice of 1 lemon

¼ cup chopped fresh parsley

¼ cup chopped fresh mint

½ teaspoon sea salt

¼ teaspoon black pepper

SERVES 4 • PREP TIME: 10 MINUTES

This tabbouleh is tasty on its own, but I also love serving it with a big Greek salad with spinach, olives, Fast Feta (page 225), and hummus. Try tripling the recipe if you are going to a picnic, so there is plenty to share with friends.

In a large bowl, toss together all the ingredients until well combined.

## VARIATIONS

**CAULIFLOWER TABBOULEH:** For a grain-free tabbouleh, replace the quinoa with cauliflower grated into cauliflower "rice" or finely chopped.

**CITRUS TABBOULEH:** Replace the lemon juice with orange or grapefruit juice for a twist. Include ½ teaspoon grated zest from the orange or grapefruit.

**TIP:** *To grate broccoli or cauliflower, use either a box grater or the grater attachment on a food processor to create a rice-like texture. To achieve the same results with the traditional food-processor blade, simply pulse until you reach the desired texture.*

# Seared Polenta with Sautéed Greens

**GF** **NF** **SF** **30**

1 tablespoon plus 1 teaspoon olive oil, divided

¼ (18-ounce) tube prepared polenta or ¼ batch polenta (page 84), cut into 4 (½-inch) slices

1 bunch Swiss chard, stemmed and roughly chopped

¼ teaspoon sea salt

¼ teaspoon black pepper

**TIP:** *Polenta can stick to the pan, so getting the perfect sear is an act of patience. You will be tempted to check it or flip it, but be patient and wait at least 4 minutes. Gently nudge it with your spatula, and if it doesn't budge, wait 2 more minutes, and then it should be ready to flip. I guarantee that your first time trying this you will think it's burning, but it really takes a while for it to sear. You have to let it release itself from the pan—and that takes time.*

SERVES 2 • PREP TIME: 5 MINUTES • COOK TIME: 15 MINUTES

I love polenta so much that if I make more than I need, I will just eat it and eat it and eat it. Making a small portion like this for me and my partner allows me to completely satisfy our appetites without overdoing it with more polenta than we need for a sensible meal. Of course, if you are feeding your entire family or a group of friends, simply double or triple this recipe.

**1.** Heat 1 tablespoon of oil in a large skillet over medium-high heat. Let the oil get very hot, then add the polenta slices and sear for 4 to 6 minutes. Flip and sear for an additional 4 to 6 minutes, until lightly browned. You might have to do this in more than one batch, depending on the size of your skillet. Add more oil as needed.

**2.** Transfer the polenta rounds to a plate and cover with an inverted plate to keep warm.

**3.** Lower the heat to medium and add the remaining 1 teaspoon of oil to the same skillet. Add the chard, salt, and pepper and toss well with tongs to evenly coat. Cook for 3 minutes, or until wilted.

**4.** Divide the polenta cakes between 2 plates and top with the chard.

### VARIATIONS

**GRAINS, GREENS, AND BEANS PLATE:** This is the perfect addition to the GGB Bowl (page 28). Simply make the polenta as described and top with the GGB recipe!

**MUSHROOM RAGOUT AND POLENTA:** Complete the recipe as given. Then, in the same skillet, add another teaspoon of oil and 1 pound of a variety of mushrooms, stemmed and roughly chopped. Sauté over medium heat for 5 minutes, or until reduced in size. Whisk together ½ cup low-sodium vegetable broth, ½ teaspoon Italian seasoning, ¼ teaspoon salt, ¼ teaspoon black pepper, and 2 teaspoons cornstarch. Slowly add this mixture to the skillet and stir for 4 minutes, or until thickened. Spoon the mushroom mixture over the polenta and greens.

# Polenta Tots

1 (18-ounce) tube prepared polenta
   or 1 batch polenta (page 84),
   cut into tot-size pieces

Nonstick cooking spray

½ teaspoon garlic powder

¼ teaspoon sea salt

2 pinches black pepper

Ketchup or other dipping sauce,
   for serving (optional)

SERVES 6 TO 8 • PREP TIME: 5 MINUTES •
COOK TIME: 25 MINUTES

Tater tots are a classic, and while I still love potatoes, I find satisfaction in grabbing a tube of premade polenta at the grocery store or using some I have already made and cutting it up into tot-size pieces. My favorite is the Parmesan Polenta Tots variation, but make all three and choose your own winner.

**1.** Preheat the oven to 450°F. Line a baking sheet with parchment paper.

**2.** Spread the polenta tots in an even layer on the prepared baking sheet and spray them with nonstick cooking spray.

**3.** In a small bowl, mix together the garlic powder, salt, and pepper and sprinkle half of the mixture on the tots from 8 to 12 inches above, to evenly cover all pieces. Bake for 14 minutes. Flip the tots with a spatula, spray again, season with the remaining garlic powder mixture, and bake for an additional 12 minutes, or until browned and crispy.

**4.** Serve with ketchup or your preferred dipping sauce.

### VARIATIONS

**PARMESAN POLENTA TOTS:** Add ¼ cup Walnut Parmesan (page 230) when seasoning the tots. Serve with Magnificent Marinara (page 231) for dipping.

**TRUFFLE POLENTA TOTS:** Instead of nonstick cooking spray, invest in some high-quality truffle oil. Drizzle 2 teaspoons over the polenta on the prepared baking sheet. Toss with a spatula, then season and bake as indicated in the recipe.

**TIP:** *Sometimes polenta can take a while to brown or crisp up, even at 450°F. If you're having trouble achieving crisping after the indicated baking time, broil the tots for 2 to 4 minutes, toss, and broil again for 2 to 4 more minutes, until you get your desired crispiness. Be mindful that everyone's broil setting is different, and these can go from crispy perfection to burnt in the blink of an eye.*

# Cheese Grits

2 cups unsweetened soy or
   almond milk

2 cups water

1½ teaspoons sea salt

1 cup stone-ground cornmeal

¼ cup vegan butter

½ teaspoon black pepper

1 cup Easy Cheese Sauce (page 224) or
   store-bought vegan cheddar shreds

SERVES 4 TO 6 · PREP TIME: 5 MINUTES ·
COOK TIME: 25 MINUTES

I grew up in Michigan, but my father is a born and raised Southern gent from Alabama. I remember visiting my family down South on several occasions and being hesitant to eat black-eyed peas and grits (not to mention being terrified of my no-nonsense Southern granny, may she rest in peace). As I grew up, I learned to appreciate the differences in Northern and Southern cuisine, and also to veganize some of those classic dishes. This recipe is for my dad.

**1.** In a large saucepot, bring the milk, water, and salt to a boil over medium-high heat. Gradually add the cornmeal while whisking constantly.

**2.** Reduce the heat to low, cover, and simmer for 20 to 25 minutes, until the mixture is creamy, whisking every 3 to 4 minutes to prevent the grits from sticking or forming lumps.

**3.** Remove from the heat and whisk in the butter and pepper. Once the butter is melted, gradually whisk in the cheese, a little at a time. Serve immediately.

### VARIATIONS

**FRESH HERB GRITS:** Omit the cheese. Stir in 1 tablespoon minced fresh rosemary and 1 tablespoon minced fresh thyme, and garnish with chopped fresh chives and freshly ground black pepper.

**SOUTHERN BREAKFAST PLATTER:** Serve this up alongside Sheet-Pan Black Bean Home Fries (page 59) and Scrappy Scrambler (page 138) for a complete breakfast platter!

**TIP:** *Sometimes finding a bag labeled "polenta" in the supermarket is tough, but this recipe proves that you can use simple stone-ground cornmeal to achieve your polenta goals. The difference between that and a bag labeled "polenta" is usually the grind, but either will work for a delicious polenta dish.*

# Creamy Parmesan Polenta

GF 30

4 cups water

1 teaspoon sea salt

1 cup yellow cornmeal or polenta

1 cup Walnut Parmesan (page 230) or
   store-bought vegan Parmesan

2 tablespoons vegan butter

SERVES 6 TO 8 • PREP TIME: 2 MINUTES •
COOK TIME: 25 MINUTES

With polenta, it all comes down to how it is prepared. You will notice that this recipe isn't much different from the recipe at the beginning of this chapter for basic polenta (page 84). The only difference is that the basic one goes into the fridge to set so it can be used for grilling and searing. This version can be enjoyed immediately, and brings much comfort and warmth to the dinner table.

1. In a large saucepot, bring the water to a boil over medium-high heat, then add the salt. Pour the cornmeal into the boiling water in a steady stream, whisking constantly while pouring it in.

2. Continue whisking for 3 to 5 minutes, until the polenta has thickened to a consistency where it doesn't settle back to the bottom of the pan immediately.

3. Reduce the heat to low, cover the pot, and simmer for 25 minutes for a creamy consistency. Stir vigorously every 5 minutes, making sure to scrape the sides, corners, and bottom of the pot.

4. Add the Parmesan and butter and mix thoroughly. Serve immediately or remove from the heat and let sit, covered, for 15 minutes before serving. If it sits longer, it will become thicker and less creamy.

### VARIATIONS

**POLENTA BOLOGNESE:** Top this off with a serving of Lentil Bolognese (page 78) for a very filling meal or side dish.

**SURF-AND-TURF POLENTA:** Add sautéed vegan Italian sausage slices and seared king trumpet mushrooms to the top of this polenta to wow your carnivorous guests!

**TIP:** *When you add the cornmeal to the water, whisk continuously to work the lumps out immediately, or else you will end up with a lumpy, though still delicious, finished product.*

# Mini Polenta Cheese Pizzas

1 tablespoon olive oil, or more
if needed

½ (18-ounce) tube prepared polenta
or ½ batch polenta (page 84),
cut into ½-inch slices

1 cup Magnificent Marinara (page 231)
or store-bought marinara

1 cup Easy Cheese Sauce–Mozzarella
variation (page 224) or store-bought
vegan mozzarella shreds

¼ cup Walnut Parmesan (page 230)
or store-bought vegan Parmesan,
for garnish (optional)

Chopped fresh basil, for garnish
(optional)

**SERVES 6 • PREP TIME: 5 MINUTES • COOK TIME: 10 MINUTES**

If you haven't noticed, I like to turn anything and
everything into pizza—and why not? Pizza has everything
you need: sauce and crust! The trick to polenta crust, of
course, is getting the outside crispy before you put your
toppings on. Exercise patience when searing your polenta
(see Tip on page 101) and you can't go wrong.

**1.** Heat 1 tablespoon of oil in a large skillet over
medium-high heat. Let the oil get very hot, then add the
polenta slices and sear for 4 to 6 minutes. Flip and sear
for an additional 4 to 6 minutes, until lightly browned. You
might have to do this in more than one batch, depending
on the size of your skillet. Add more oil as needed.

**2.** Transfer the polenta rounds to a plate and dress with
marinara and cheese sauce, then garnish with Parmesan
and basil, if desired.

### VARIATIONS

**BBQ CHICKEN AND CHEDDAR PIZZAS:** Preheat the oven to
broil and line a baking sheet with parchment paper. Place
the polenta rounds on the prepared baking sheet. Top the
polenta with Basic BBQ Sauce (page 232) instead of
marinara. Add vegan chicken strips and sliced red onion,
then vegan cheddar shreds instead of cheese sauce. Broil
for 2 to 4 minutes—just enough to melt the cheese.

**VEGETABLE SUPREME PIZZAS:** Add chopped bell peppers,
onions, and mushrooms for a vegetable supreme.

**TIP:** *To get a golden bubbly finish on the top, preheat the
oven to broil and line a baking sheet with parchment paper.
Dress the polenta rounds with sauce and cheese right on
the prepared baking sheet. Broil for 2 to 4 minutes, until
just golden brown on top, then garnish with basil.*

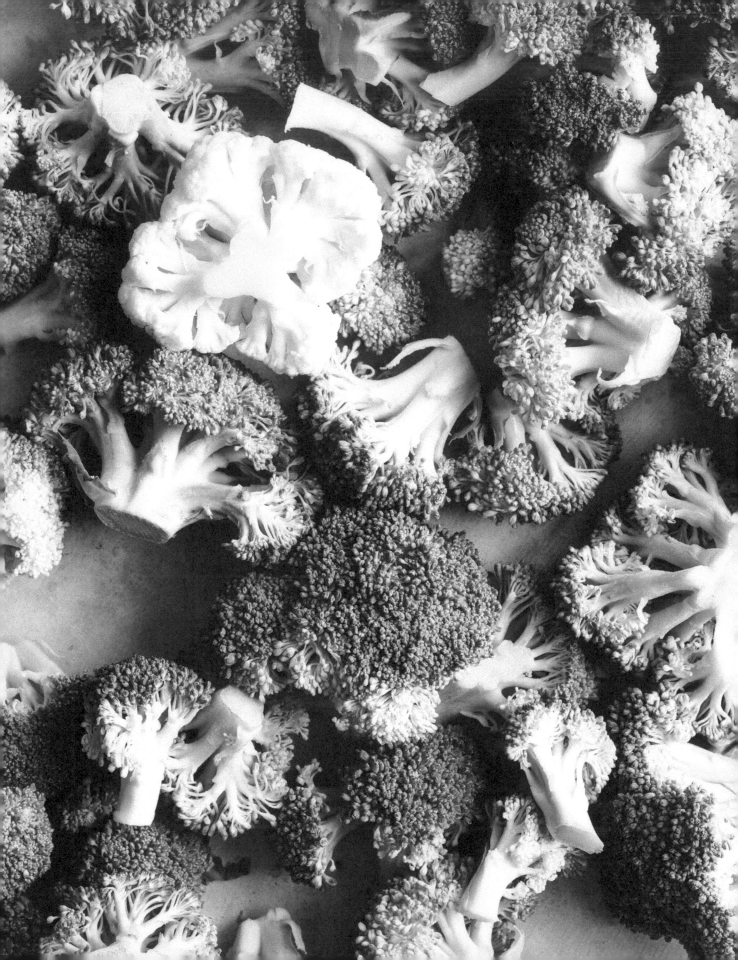

# CHAPTER 6

# Broccoli & Cauliflower

Broccoli and cauliflower are the yin and yang of vegetable land and my personal lifetime love–hate relationship. As a kid, the only way I would eat my broccoli was smothered in cheese and buried in a potato.

Make no mistake, I drew heavily on those childhood desires to deliver the following recipes. While I have grown fond of both broccoli and cauliflower as an adult, it certainly didn't happen overnight, and the struggle to finish my broccoli is certainly still an issue from time to time. But finally, I have found a place in my heart for these veggies.

Cauliflower has made huge strides in the culinary world in the last few years. From cauliflower steaks to Buffalo cauliflower wings and cauliflower–based sauces, restaurants across the country have been hopping on board the cauliflower express to deliver more healthful variations on their menus while maintaining flavor. As for broccoli—I still love it smothered in a vegan cheese sauce, but the pages ahead offer a nice mixture of these vegetables stripped down as well as dressed up, to satisfy even the pickiest of palates.

# Broccoli Slaw

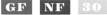

1 cup broccoli ribbons (2 to 4 broccoli stalks; see Tip)

2 cups shredded or thinly sliced purple cabbage

¼ cup Mayonnaise (page 223) or store-bought vegan mayonnaise

1 tablespoon maple syrup

1 teaspoon apple cider vinegar

½ teaspoon salt

**SERVES 4 • PREP TIME: 10 MINUTES**

This is the perfect dish to accompany any food at a summer gathering. Slip this slaw into the mix, and no need to mention it's vegan. If you are one of those people who are very specific about your slaw (tangy versus sweet), feel free to adjust the recipe with more maple syrup, vinegar, or salt, to your liking. I have found you can never please everyone when it comes to slaw, but that never stops me from trying.

In a large bowl, combine all the ingredients and toss to thoroughly mix.

### VARIATIONS

**TRADITIONAL SLAW:** Replace the purple cabbage and broccoli with green cabbage and shredded carrots.

**TROPICAL BROCCOLI SLAW:** Add 1 cup diced mango or pineapple to give this slaw a tropical twist.

**TIP:** *To make broccoli ribbons, use a potato peeler. Peel the tough outer coating away from each stalk and discard. Then use the peeler to create broccoli ribbons with the remainder of the stalk. Use the florets for Thai Roasted Broccoli (page 110) or Quinoa and Broccoli Tabbouleh (page 100).*

# Thai Roasted Broccoli

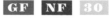

1 head broccoli, cut into florets

2 tablespoons olive oil

1 tablespoon soy sauce or
gluten-free tamari

**SERVES 4 • PREP TIME: 5 MINUTES • COOK TIME: 15 MINUTES**

If you still have ill feelings toward broccoli, roast it and your mind will be changed forever. I get into trouble roasting vegetables because when they come out of the oven and I "test" a piece . . . my test turns into a meal. It's guilt-free, except for the fact that I don't have any left to serve! I indulge in all three of these variations, but I challenge you, once you get comfortable, to spice up some broccoli with your own favorite spice combinations.

**1.** Preheat the oven to 425°F. Line a baking sheet with parchment paper.

**2.** In a large bowl, combine the broccoli, oil, and soy sauce. Toss well to combine. Spread the broccoli on the prepared baking sheet.

**3.** Roast for 10 minutes. Toss the broccoli with a spatula and roast for an additional 5 minutes, or until the edges of the florets begin to brown.

### VARIATIONS

**GARLIC AND LEMON ROASTED BROCCOLI:** Omit the soy sauce. Add 1 teaspoon garlic powder and ½ teaspoon sea salt when tossing the broccoli with the olive oil. Roast as directed, remove from the oven, and squeeze the juice of ½ lemon or more, if desired over the top of the broccoli.

**BUTTER AND PARMESAN ROASTED BROCCOLI:** Omit the olive oil and soy sauce. Toss the florets in 2 tablespoons melted vegan butter, 2 tablespoons nutritional yeast or Walnut Parmesan (page 230), and ½ teaspoon sea salt. Roast as directed.

**TIP:** *If you wish to omit the oil or butter for fewer calories, you can steam the broccoli on the stovetop until fork-tender and toss with any desired spices.*

# Cauliflower Alfredo Your Way

4 cups bite-size cauliflower florets

1½ cups unsweetened soy or almond milk

¼ cup soft or silken tofu

Juice of ½ lemon

2 tablespoons Dijon mustard

1½ teaspoons onion powder

1½ teaspoons sea salt

1 teaspoon garlic powder

¼ teaspoon black pepper, plus more for garnish (optional)

1 pound pasta of your choice, cooked

Walnut Parmesan (page 230) or store-bought vegan Parmesan, for garnish (optional)

Chopped fresh parsley, for garnish (optional)

SERVES 6 • PREP TIME: 5 MINUTES • COOK TIME: 15 MINUTES

Alfredo . . . I used to frequent a certain Italian chain restaurant when my friend Kelly worked there and order up endless breadsticks with a side of their heart attack–inducing Alfredo sauce to dip it in. Thankfully, I survived. My years of testing fate enabled me to recreate that classic sauce in a vegan version. Toss this with pasta, or use it as a dipping sauce or even a sandwich spread. Have it your way.

**1.** Steam the cauliflower for 10 to 12 minutes until fork-tender (see Tip), then transfer to a blender.

**2.** Add the milk, tofu, lemon juice, mustard, onion powder, salt, garlic powder, and pepper and blend for 1 to 2 minutes, until creamy and smooth.

**3.** Toss the cooked pasta with the sauce and divide among 6 serving bowls. Garnish with Parmesan, parsley, and more pepper, if desired.

### VARIATIONS

**BROCCOLI AND CHICKEN ALFREDO:** Add store-bought vegan grilled chicken strips and steamed broccoli to recreate a classic.

**WHITE-SAUCE PIZZA:** This sauce makes an excellent white sauce for your favorite store-bought vegan pizza dough or whole-wheat pita. For a unique twist, top the dough or pita with broccoli, corn, and diced red bell pepper, and then drizzle the veggies with Easy Cheese Sauce (page 224) or store-bought vegan mozzarella shreds. Bake at 350°F for 15 minutes. Your guests will be doing jazz hands after the last bite!

**TIP:** *If you don't have a steamer basket, submerge the cauliflower florets in boiling water instead. Cook over medium-high heat until fork-tender, about 10 minutes, then drain and transfer to the blender.*

# Stan's Cauliflower Fried Rice

`GF` `NF` `30`

1 large head cauliflower

2 tablespoons olive oil or toasted sesame oil, divided

1 onion, chopped

1 (8-ounce) package baby bella or white button mushrooms, stemmed and sliced

3 garlic cloves, minced

1 cup frozen peas

1 cup julienned, shredded, or thinly sliced carrot

1 cup shredded or finely sliced purple cabbage

3 tablespoons soy sauce or gluten-free tamari

¼ teaspoon sea salt

¼ teaspoon black pepper

2 scallions, thinly sliced

Sriracha sauce, for garnish (optional)

**TIP:** *While julienning carrots is super pretty and adds flair to your meal, don't stress yourself out with perfect cuts. If you are short on time, I highly recommend buying a bag of shredded carrots to cut down on the prep, or just grating or thinly slicing the carrots—whatever is easiest for you.*

SERVES 4 TO 6 • PREP TIME: 15 MINUTES • COOK TIME: 15 MINUTES

One of my private chef clients is in love with this cauliflower fried rice—so much so that I decided to name it after him! While classic fried rice is delicious, it's nice to know there is an alternative that is less carb-heavy but still packs the same amount of flavor. My hope is that you find some creative freedom with this recipe; try it once as is and then feel free to add your favorite veggies to it.

**1.** Grate the cauliflower in a food processor with the grating disk or on the large holes of a box or handheld grater. You should end up with about 4 cups of cauliflower "rice."

**2.** Heat 1 tablespoon of oil in a large skillet over medium heat. Add the onion and mushrooms and sauté for about 5 minutes, until the mushrooms are soft and reduced in size. Add the garlic and cook for 1 minute, or until fragrant.

**3.** Add the remaining 1 tablespoon of oil and the grated cauliflower. Mix well and cook for 2 minutes. Mix in the peas, carrot, cabbage, and soy sauce and cook for about 4 minutes, stirring occasionally, until the cauliflower rice is starting to get tender but is still firm. Add the salt and pepper and stir to combine.

**4.** Portion onto plates and garnish with the scallions. Drizzle with sriracha if you like some heat.

## VARIATIONS

**TOFU EGG FRIED RICE:** This will require Himalayan black salt (kala namak), which is found at most health food stores and online. Add ½ teaspoon of the black salt to a ½ (14-ounce) block extra-firm tofu that has been drained and crumbled. Add the tofu to the recipe when you add the garlic.

**PINEAPPLE FRIED CAULIFLOWER RICE:** Cut a pineapple in half lengthwise and scoop out the flesh. Cut into bite-size pieces and add 1½ cups to the skillet when you add the peas, carrot, and cabbage. To impress your guests, serve the rice in the hollowed-out pineapple shells.

# Kentucky Baked Cauliflower

Nonstick cooking spray

1 cup unsweetened soy or almond milk

1 tablespoon apple cider vinegar

1 cup all-purpose flour

1 tablespoon paprika

1½ teaspoons sea salt

1 teaspoon dried oregano

1 teaspoon dried parsley

½ teaspoon dried thyme

½ teaspoon onion powder

½ teaspoon garlic powder

½ teaspoon black pepper

1 head cauliflower, cut into
    medium florets

**TIP:** *Use one hand to dip the cauliflower pieces in the liquid and the other hand for coating in the dry mixture, to create a seamless flow and a mess-free dredging station.*

SERVES 4 • PREP TIME: 10 MINUTES • COOK TIME: 30 MINUTES

We are in a wonderful world when you can switch out fast-food chicken for a super satisfying, crispy, perfectly spiced, and—dare I say—finger-lickin' good cauliflower option! I love this baked cauliflower so much; it goes great with mashed potatoes and gravy and fills me up every time.

1. Preheat the oven to 450°F. Line a baking sheet with parchment paper and coat with nonstick cooking spray.

2. In a small bowl, whisk together the milk and vinegar.

3. In a medium bowl, whisk together the flour, paprika, salt, oregano, parsley, thyme, onion powder, garlic powder, and pepper.

4. Dip the cauliflower pieces into the milk mixture and then transfer them one by one to the medium bowl and coat with the flour mixture. Once each piece is coated, transfer it to the prepared baking sheet. Spray the coated cauliflower pieces with nonstick cooking spray.

5. Bake for 15 minutes, then flip the cauliflower, spray again, and bake for an additional 15 minutes, or until darker in color and crunchy.

## VARIATIONS

**COUNTRY BAKED CAULIFLOWER STEAK:** Instead of florets, cut the head of cauliflower lengthwise through the core into 4 "steaks." Continue with the recipe as written. Smother the steaks with Country Sausage Gravy (page 229) to serve.

**KENTUCKY BAKED BBQ CAULIFLOWER SALAD:** Instead of medium florets, cut the cauliflower into bite-size florets and continue with the recipe as written. While it's baking, in a large bowl toss together 1 head romaine lettuce, chopped, 1 tomato, chopped, and ½ cup shredded carrots. Divide the salad among 4 bowls. Toss the baked cauliflower bites with Basic BBQ Sauce (page 232) and divide among the 4 salads. Drizzle with Unhidden Valley Ranch Dressing (page 221).

# Roasted Mexican–Spiced Cauliflower

   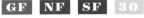

GF   NF   SF   30

1 head cauliflower, cut into bite-size florets

½ cup frozen or fresh corn kernels

4 garlic cloves, sliced

2 tablespoons olive oil

1 tablespoon Taco Seasoning (page 219) or store-bought taco seasoning

2 scallions, thinly sliced, for garnish

SERVES 4 TO 6 • PREP TIME: 5 MINUTES • COOK TIME: 25 MINUTES

Roasted cauliflower has become a go-to for me in the last couple of years. It is extremely satisfying and also fun to play around with using your favorite seasonings on it. It's great as a side dish or entrée, served over greens or rice (or both!), or just to snack on when you have the craving to munch.

1. Preheat the oven to 425°F. Line a baking sheet with parchment paper.

2. In a large bowl toss together the cauliflower, corn, garlic, oil, and taco seasoning. Spread the cauliflower mixture evenly on the prepared baking sheet.

3. Bake for 15 minutes, toss with a spatula, and bake for an additional 10 minutes, or until the cauliflower has gotten darker and browned slightly on the edges. Serve garnished with the scallions.

## VARIATIONS

**CAULIFLOWER POPCORN:** Omit the corn, garlic, and taco seasoning. Cut the florets into popcorn-size pieces. Toss with the olive oil and season with salt and pepper. Bake at 425°F for 10 minutes, toss, and bake for an additional 10 minutes, or until tender but still crisp on the outside. Enjoy while you watch your favorite movie.

**ROASTED CAULIFLOWER SKEWERS:** Omit the corn and garlic. Toss the cauliflower with the olive oil and taco seasoning and roast as directed, cool, and thread onto skewers with baby bella mushrooms, cherry tomatoes, red onion chunks, and bell pepper pieces. Heat the olive oil in a large skillet and sear all sides of each skewer. Great for parties!

**TIP:** *An easy approach to cutting cauliflower is to cut the head in half and then carve the stalk out. From there, the florets break off easily, and you can trim them to size.*

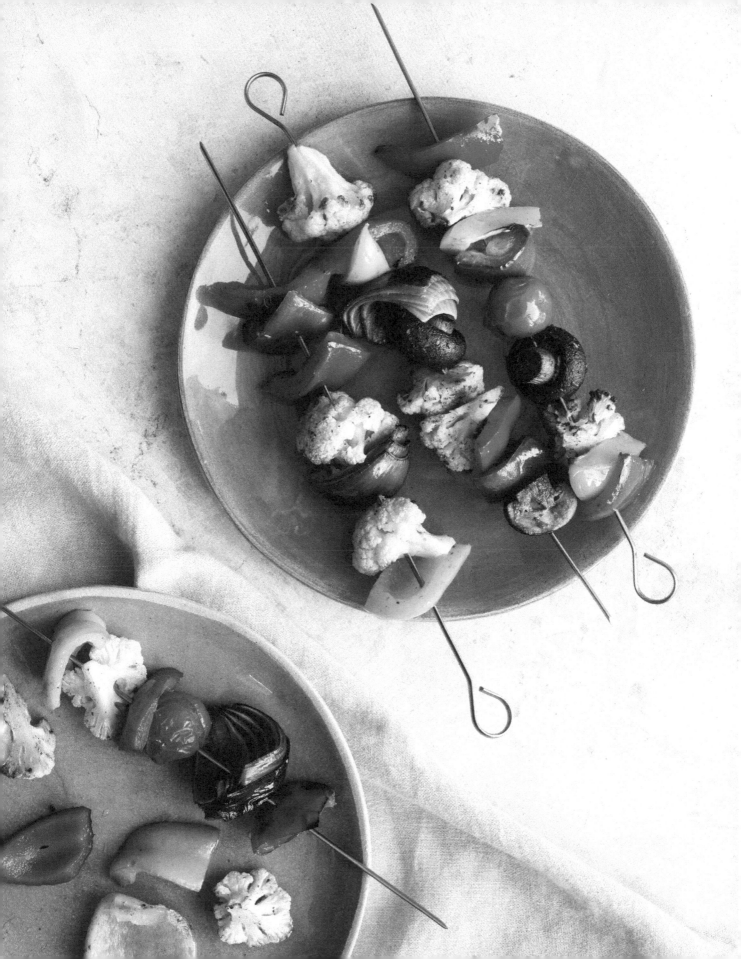

# Roasted Sweet-and-Sour Cauliflower

1 head cauliflower, cut into bite-size florets

2 tablespoons olive oil

¾ cup organic cane sugar

⅔ cup water

⅓ cup apple cider vinegar or white vinegar

1 tablespoon ketchup

¼ cup soy sauce or gluten-free tamari

2 tablespoons cornstarch

4 cups cooked brown rice

2 scallions, chopped, for garnish (optional)

White sesame seeds, for garnish (optional)

**TIP:** *Cut the cauliflower pieces the same size for even roasting.*

SERVES 4 • PREP TIME: 5 MINUTES • COOK TIME: 25 MINUTES

I struggle a bit with not easily being able to order Chinese take-out anymore. Things that should be vegan just aren't, mostly because of the addition of fish sauce. In this version of sweet and sour, it's all about a simple sauce paired with a vegetable and a grain. I love to throw this together when I have a head of cauliflower lying around that I've been meaning to do something with.

**1.** Preheat the oven to 450°F. Line a baking sheet with parchment paper.

**2.** In a large bowl, toss the cauliflower florets with the oil and spread out on the prepared baking sheet. Roast for 15 minutes, toss with a spatula, and roast for an additional 10 minutes, or until fork-tender.

**3.** While the cauliflower is roasting, mix together the sugar, water, vinegar, and ketchup in a large skillet. Bring the mixture to a boil over medium-high heat, then reduce to a simmer.

**4.** In a small bowl, whisk together the soy sauce and cornstarch to create a slurry. Slowly stir the slurry into the sauce until well combined and the sauce thickens, 2 to 4 minutes.

**5.** When the cauliflower is finished, transfer to the skillet and toss well to coat with the sauce.

**6.** Divide the rice among 4 bowls, top with the cauliflower, and garnish with scallions and sesame seeds, if desired.

## VARIATIONS

**TRADITIONAL SWEET-AND-SOUR CAULIFLOWER:** Add 1 onion and 1 green bell pepper, both diced, to the baking sheet with the cauliflower for the last 10 minutes of baking, for a more traditional sweet-and-sour dish with vegetables.

**SWEET-AND-SOUR CHICKEN:** Omit the cauliflower. Prepare vegan chicken strips according to the package directions and dress with the sauce.

# Mom's Creamy Broccoli and Rice Bake

**GF**

2 cups cooked brown rice

1 (12-ounce) bag frozen broccoli florets, chopped, or 2 cups chopped fresh broccoli florets

½ cup chopped onion

1 celery stalk, thinly sliced

1 batch Easy Cheese Sauce (page 224)

SERVES 6 TO 8 • PREP TIME: 10 MINUTES • COOK TIME: 40 MINUTES

When I was a kid, it wasn't a holiday without my mom making this casserole. Her version consisted of all the dairy she could get her hands on in the mid-Michigan area. I have been trying to replicate that super-simple dish of ooey-gooey, creamy deliciousness for the last 10 years, and I'm confident that I finally did it. I hope this dish finds a spot at your holiday table.

**1.** Preheat the oven to 425°F.

**2.** In a large bowl, mix together the rice, broccoli, onion, celery, and cheese sauce. Transfer to a 2-quart or 8-inch-square baking dish.

**3.** Bake for 40 minutes, or until the top has started to brown slightly.

## VARIATIONS

**TOTS 'N' BROCCOLI CASSEROLE:** Omit the rice and add 2 cups frozen tater tots. Bake the casserole for 30 to 40 minutes, being mindful not to burn the tops of the tater tots, as different brands will cook at different times.

**BACON CRUST CASSEROLE:** Top with crushed potato chips in the last 10 minutes of baking. Remove from the oven and sprinkle on chopped Portobello Bacon (page 185).

**TIP:** *The Easy Cheese Sauce provides the perfect substitute for the canned "cream of" soups my mom used to use in different variations of this recipe. Unfortunately, subbing store-bought vegan cheese shreds won't work here. But you can substitute Heidi Ho Cheeze sauce, if need be, found at some grocery stores and most natural food stores.*

# Broccoli and Cheese Twice-Baked Potatoes

**GF**

2 large russet potatoes, washed and halved

1 teaspoon olive oil

Sea salt

2 cups chopped broccoli florets

1 cup Easy Cheese Sauce (page 224), divided

SERVES 4 • PREP TIME: 5 MINUTES • COOK TIME: 40 MINUTES

Wendy's drive-through had my number growing up: that quick yet decadent Frosty, the chili that was perfect for a cold Michigan winter evening, and that gosh darn baked potato! I started throwing this potato recipe together a couple of years back, when I had that specific craving, and I'm happy to say it fed my nostalgic curiosity and satiated both my hunger and taste buds.

**1.** Preheat the oven to 425°F. Line a baking sheet with parchment paper.

**2.** Rub the potato halves all over with the oil and place on the prepared baking sheet, cut-sides down. Sprinkle with salt. Bake for 25 minutes, or until just fork-tender. Remove from the oven and let cool for 15 minutes.

**3.** Scoop out the insides of the potatoes and transfer them to a medium bowl. Be careful not to tear the potato skins as you do this. Add the broccoli and ¾ cup cheese sauce to the potato insides and mix until well combined.

**4.** Divide the mixture among the hollowed-out potato halves, drizzle with the remaining ¼ cup of cheese sauce, and sprinkle with salt. Bake for 15 minutes, until the drizzled cheese begins to brown.

**VARIATIONS**

**DELUXE TWICE-BAKED POTATOES:** Top with Sour Cream (page 222), Portobello Bacon (page 185), and chopped scallions after the final bake.

**CURRY CHICKPEA TWICE-BAKED POTATOES:** Omit the broccoli and Easy Cheese Sauce. Add 1 (15-ounce) can chickpeas, rinsed and drained, 2 tablespoons olive oil, 2 tablespoons curry powder, and ½ teaspoon sea salt to the potato insides. Mix until well combined and divide among the hollowed-out potato halves. Bake for 15 minutes.

**TIP:** *A melon baller is very helpful for scooping out the insides of the potatoes.*

# Broccoli and Black Bean Tostadas

  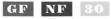

**GF** **NF** **30**

1½ cups chopped broccoli florets

1 (15-ounce) can black beans, rinsed and drained

½ cup halved cherry tomatoes

½ cup stemmed and diced baby bella or white button mushrooms

2 tablespoons olive oil, or more as needed, divided

2 teaspoons soy sauce or gluten-free tamari

1 teaspoon garlic powder

1 teaspoon onion powder

4 (6-inch) corn tortillas

Sriracha sauce

Sour Cream (page 222) or store-bought vegan sour cream, for garnish (optional)

Chopped fresh cilantro, for garnish (optional)

**SERVES 4 · PREP TIME: 10 MINUTES · COOK TIME: 20 MINUTES**

Foods you eat with your hands are the best! And tostadas make a fun DIY dinner night with the family. I suggest pulling this sheet-pan recipe together with some fixin's on the side, such as vegan cheese shreds, shredded lettuce, various hot sauces, rice, and so on, to let everyone play with making their own variations.

**1.** Preheat the oven to 425°F. Line a baking sheet with parchment paper.

**2.** In a large bowl, mix together the broccoli, beans, tomatoes, mushrooms, 1 tablespoon olive oil, soy sauce, garlic powder, and onion powder. Spread out the mixture on the prepared baking sheet. Bake for 10 minutes, toss with a spatula, and bake for an additional 5 to 10 minutes, until the beans start to split and the broccoli is fork-tender.

**3.** While the mixture is baking, heat the remaining 1 tablespoon of olive oil in a medium skillet over medium-high heat. Lightly fry each tortilla on both sides until golden brown, adding more oil as needed.

**4.** Divide the baked mixture among the 4 crispy tortillas and gently smash some of the beans down on the tortillas so the mixture sticks. Drizzle with sriracha. Add some sour cream and cilantro, if desired.

### VARIATIONS

**BLACK BEAN CAULIFLOWER TOSTADAS:** Replace the broccoli with chopped cauliflower florets.

**KALE-LUPAS:** Omit the entire broccoli mixture. Fry the tortillas as directed and top with store-bought vegan refried beans and sautéed kale and corn. Garnish with salsa and chopped scallions.

**TIP:** *Sprinkle a drop of water into the oil in the pan; when it pops, the oil is hot enough to start frying the tortillas.*

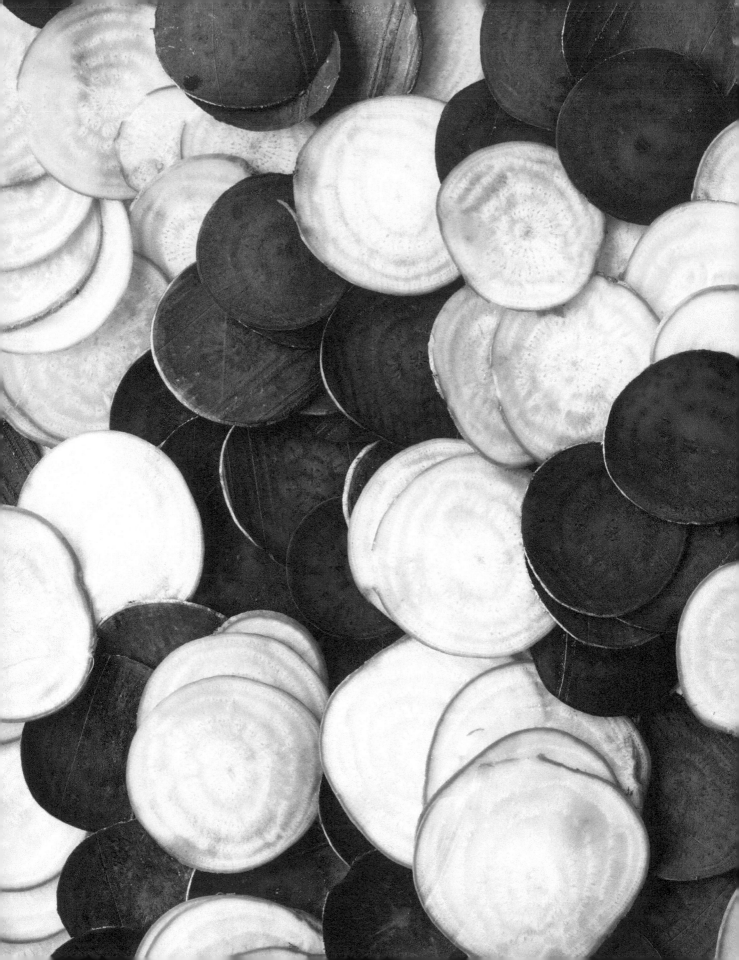

# CHAPTER 7

# Root Vegetables

Root vegetables are delicious and are considered to be among the most nutrient-dense vegetables. There are a ton of root vegetables, but some of the most common are daikon, carrot, yucca (cassava), yam, beet, parsnip, potato, turnip, rutabaga, celery root, horseradish, radish. . . .

This chapter focuses on some root vegetables that are easiest to find at your standard supermarket. Most root vegetables are available year round. However, their peak season is fall through spring, with the exception of beets, which are best summer through fall. Selecting a root vegetable is unlike selecting any other piece of produce in the store, because with root vegetables, the harder the better.

I encourage you to get comfortable with the recipes in the next several pages and then start to explore the wondrous world of root veggies beyond these pages. For example, one of my favorite dishes that I have found on my travels is a rutabaga fondue from the restaurant Vedge in Philadelphia. While I tried to whip up a version for this book, it wasn't necessarily true to the title "simple"—but I had to mention it so you have an idea of just how inventive and creative you can be. And by all means, if you find yourself in Philly, get yourself a reservation at Vedge and get that fondue! But for now, start with these root vegetables at home.

# Berry Beetsicle Smoothie

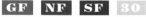

½ cup peeled and diced beets

½ cup frozen raspberries

1 frozen banana

1 tablespoon maple syrup

1 cup unsweetened soy or almond milk

**SERVES 1 · PREP TIME: 3 MINUTES**

Unicorns are all the rage these days. If you feel so inclined, you can skip right to the unicorn variation on this smoothie with a dollop of Coconut Whipped Cream (page 202) and some rainbow sprinkles. It has that beautiful pink color required of all things unicorn. This recipe is quick, healthful, and so beautiful that I feel like Wonder Woman when I drink it!

Combine all the ingredients in a blender and blend until smooth.

### VARIATIONS

**UNICORN SMOOTHIE:** Make this smoothie and set aside in the refrigerator. Rinse out the blender and combine 1 more frozen banana with ½ cup unsweetened soy or almond milk and 2 blueberries (yes, just 2). Blend until smooth; it should be blue. Pour half of the Berry Beetsicle Smoothie into a drinking glass or mason jar, then the blueberry mixture, then the rest of the beetsicle. Top with Coconut Whipped Cream (page 202) and vegan rainbow sprinkles.

**CITRUS-BEET SMOOTHIE:** Omit the milk and raspberries. Add ½ cup peeled and chopped orange and 1 cup orange juice.

**TIP:** *There's no way of getting around it, beets are a beautiful red-producing machine, and this means on your hands. It's worth it to invest in a box of rubber gloves from the dollar store when you are a starting a love affair with beets!*

# Fancy-Free Beet Tartare with Creamy Pine Nut Ricotta

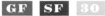  

1 pound beets, peeled and cut into ¼-inch cubes

1 teaspoon olive oil

½ teaspoon red wine vinegar

2 pinches plus ¼ teaspoon sea salt, divided

Pinch black pepper

1 scallion, minced

¾ cup pine nuts

½ cup water

½ teaspoon garlic powder

SERVES 4 · PREP TIME: 15 MINUTES

Tartare doesn't have to be a pretentious dish at an upscale restaurant. It can be a fun, tasty, easy, and colorful appetizer served up at a dinner party with your friends. This tartare is a deconstructed version; feel free to mold the beets into a disk with a cookie cutter, although it's not necessary. The presentation is so colorful and the flavor combination with the sauce is a win-win, no matter what the shape.

**1.** In a large bowl, toss together the beets, oil, vinegar, 2 pinches sea salt, pepper, and scallion until well combined.

**2.** In a blender, combine the pine nuts, water, garlic powder, remaining ¼ teaspoon sea salt and blend. The texture will not be silky smooth, but more like a chunky ricotta texture.

**3.** Divide the sauce among 4 appetizer plates and top with the beets.

### VARIATIONS

**WATERMELON-AVOCADO TARTARE:** Omit the beets. Mix 1 cup watermelon cubes with ½ avocado, cubed. Lightly toss with the dressing ingredients to coat, then continue with the recipe as written.

**ROASTED GOLD AND RED TARTARE:** Take it down to ½ pound red beets. Add ½ pound golden beets. Omit the scallion and continue with the recipe as written.

**TIP:** *To get consistent cuts with your beets, first cut ¼-inch-thick slices. Stack 3 slices on top of one another and cut into ¼-inch-thick sticks. Then cut the sticks the other way to make ¼-inch cubes. Repeat with the remaining beets, stacking only 3 at a time to maintain consistency.*

# Garlic–Parmesan Turnip Crisps

2 large turnips, peeled and cut into ⅛-inch slices

1 tablespoon olive oil

1 tablespoon Walnut Parmesan (page 230) or store-bought vegan Parmesan

½ teaspoon garlic powder

¼ teaspoon sea salt

SERVES 2 • PREP TIME: 5 MINUTES • COOK TIME: 25 MINUTES

I love a good potato chip, but what about a chip that is good for you? Enter the turnip. The turnip has had a seat at the weird kids' table at lunch for years. (I can say that; I sat at that table.) A little olive oil and seasoning gives this boring vegetable a crispy charm that will be gobbled up.

1. Preheat the oven to 400°F. Line a baking sheet with parchment paper.

2. In a large bowl, toss the turnip slices with the oil, Parmesan, garlic powder, and salt.

3. Spread the turnips evenly on the baking sheet and bake for 15 minutes. Flip and bake for an additional 10 minutes, or until some of the edges are curling up and golden brown.

### VARIATIONS

**SALT AND VINEGAR TURNIP CRISPS:** Omit the Parmesan and garlic powder. Add 2 teaspoons apple cider vinegar and an additional ¼ teaspoon salt (½ teaspoon salt total).

**SALT AND PEPPER TURNIP CRISPS:** Omit the Parmesan and garlic powder. Add ½ teaspoon black pepper and an additional ¼ teaspoon salt (½ teaspoon salt total).

TIP: *A mandoline is the perfect tool for achieving uniformly thin slices, or a slicing attachment on a food processor. But if you don't have either, you can easily slice these up with a good knife.*

# Buttered Carrot Noodles with Kale

**GF** **NF** 30

¼ cup vegan butter

½ cup chopped onion

1 pound carrots, peeled and sliced with a potato peeler or spiralizer

1 bunch lacinato kale, stemmed and thinly sliced

¼ cup chopped fresh parsley

¼ teaspoon sea salt

½ teaspoon black pepper

**SERVES 2 TO 4 • PREP TIME: 10 MINUTES • COOK TIME: 10 MINUTES**

Making noodles with your vegetables is fun. You can quickly and easily make beautiful carrot ribbons with a good old-fashioned potato peeler, no fancy spiralizer required. But if you happen to have a spiralizer, noodle those carrots up into spaghetti-like strands, as you can see on the opposite page. The veggie pasta-bilities are endless. See what I did there?

**1.** In a large skillet, melt the butter over medium heat. Add the onion and sauté for 3 minutes, or until soft.

**2.** Add the carrots and sauté for 3 minutes more, tossing in the butter until the carrots begin to brown on the edges. Add the kale and sauté for an additional 2 minutes, or until wilted.

**3.** Mix in the parsley, salt, and pepper.

### VARIATIONS

**MOROCCAN-STYLE CARROT NOODLES WITH KALE:** Just before adding the carrots, add ½ teaspoon ground cumin and ¼ teaspoon ground cinnamon to the onion mixture and toss to coat the onion. Add ½ cup raisins when adding the carrots.

**MAPLE-GLAZED CARROT NOODLES WITH KALE:** Use just 2 tablespoons butter, and add 2 tablespoons maple syrup when adding the carrots.

**TIP:** *Carrots are available at the supermarket in a 1-pound bag, making them an easy grab at the grocery store.*

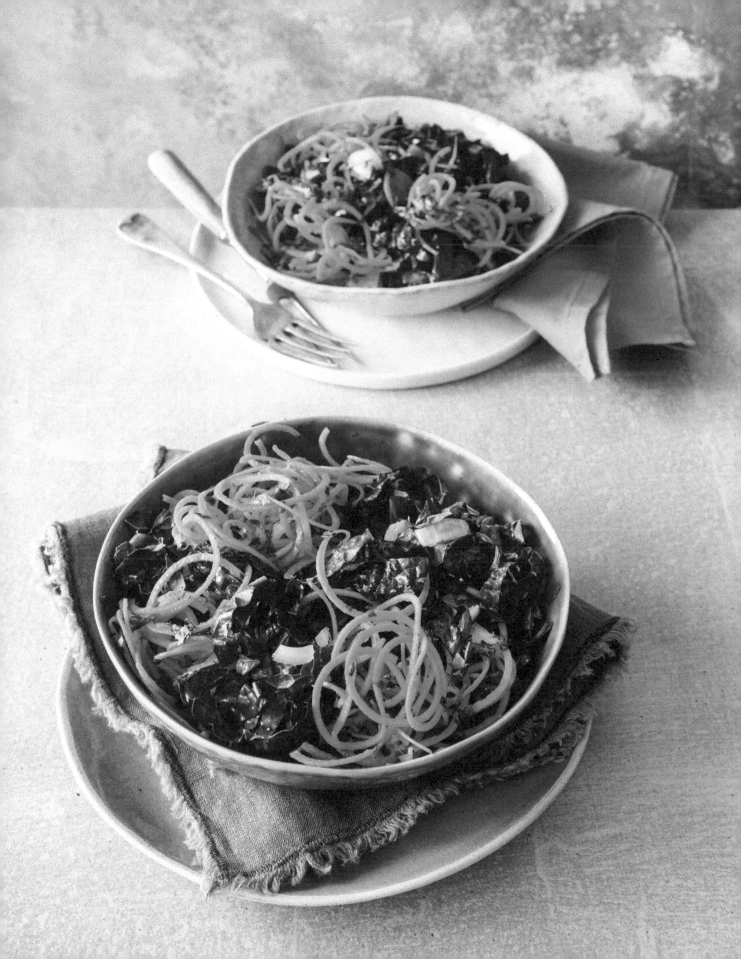

# Roasted Rosemary Potatoes

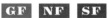

**GF**  **NF**  **SF**

1½ pounds baby red potatoes, halved

2 tablespoons olive oil

3 garlic cloves, minced

1 tablespoon minced fresh rosemary

¾ teaspoon sea salt

SERVES 4 TO 6 • PREP TIME: 5 MINUTES •
COOK TIME: 30 MINUTES

Potatoes should have their own food group as far as I'm concerned. They are so versatile and satisfying, I would be thrilled to eat them with every single meal. This recipe is simple and adds a lovely fragrance to your kitchen when cooking. It makes for a delightful side dish for any meal, or served on top of a big bowl of greens.

**1.** Preheat the oven to 425°F. Line a baking sheet with parchment paper.

**2.** In a large bowl, toss the potatoes with the oil, garlic, rosemary, and salt until well combined.

**3.** Spread the potatoes evenly on the prepared baking sheet and bake for 15 minutes. Toss with a spatula and bake for an additional 15 minutes, or until golden brown.

### VARIATIONS

**ROASTED GARLIC AND PARMESAN POTATOES:** Replace the rosemary with 2 tablespoons Walnut Parmesan (page 230).

**ROASTED TACO POTATOES:** Replace the rosemary with 2 tablespoons Taco Seasoning (page 219).

**TIP:** *Cut back on the amount of oil if you want to reduce the fat content. While it adds a richness and depth to the flavor, it's not vital to the dish if you are watching those calories.*

# Classic Mashed Potatoes

GF NF 30

3 pounds Yukon gold potatoes, peeled and cubed

Sea salt

¼ cup vegan butter

¼ cup unsweetened soy or almond milk

Freshly ground black pepper

SERVES 4 TO 6 • PREP TIME: 10 MINUTES • COOK TIME: 20 MINUTES

Surely you remember the Thanksgiving episode of *Friends* where Monica had to make mashed potatoes three ways: with lumps for Ross, whipped with peas and onions for Phoebe, and tater tots for Joey. The best part about a classic recipe is that you can take it from here and do whatever you like. If you have friends with specific needs on Thanksgiving, or any other day of the year, this recipe will get you started off strong.

**1.** Put the potatoes in a large stockpot, cover with water, salt the water generously, cover, and bring to a boil over medium-high heat. Cook the potatoes for 12 to 18 minutes, until fork-tender. The potatoes should break when poked with a fork. Drain and return to the stockpot.

**2.** Add the butter and milk. Mash with any type of masher you have on hand that does the job. Season with salt and pepper.

**VARIATIONS**

**CAULIFLOWER MASH:** Use only 2 potatoes. Add them to the pot of boiling water with 1 head cauliflower, cut into florets. Boil until fork-tender, drain, and transfer to a food processor. You may have to do this in two batches, depending on the size of your food processor. Add only 2 tablespoons vegan butter. If you feel you need more liquid to get the texture you desire, start by adding 1 tablespoon of milk at a time. Be careful with liquid, as this can easily go from a decadent mash to a soup. Transfer to a large bowl and season with salt and pepper to taste.

**SWEET POTATO MASH:** Use 3 pounds sweet potatoes instead of the Yukon gold potatoes.

**TIP:** *I have a hand potato masher, and that works just fine. But you might be fancy and get a potato ricer. I leave some lumps for a rustic appeal, but again, live your life. You do you—mash these up your way.*

# One Sheet, Turnip the Beet!

NF SF

1 pound turnips, peeled and cut into 1-inch pieces

1 pound beets, peeled and cut into 1-inch pieces

1 onion, roughly chopped into large pieces

2 tablespoons olive oil

¾ teaspoon sea salt

½ teaspoon black pepper

½ cup French's fried onions

¼ cup chopped fresh parsley

SERVES 4 TO 6 · PREP TIME: 10 MINUTES · COOK TIME: 35 MINUTES

Roasted vegetables always bring a warm and comforting feeling to the dinner table. Not only that, they are easy to toss together and throw into the oven while you go about making the rest of the dinner. Mix one of these variations together with ease and enjoy.

**1.** Preheat the oven to 425°F. Line a baking sheet with parchment paper.

**2.** In a large bowl, toss together the turnips, beets, onion, oil, salt, and pepper until evenly coated.

**3.** Spread the mixture on the prepared baking sheet and bake for 20 minutes. Toss with a spatula and bake for 10 additional minutes. Toss again, sprinkle on the fried onions and parsley, and bake for 5 more minutes, or until the turnips and beets are fork-tender.

### VARIATIONS

**TURNIP THE BEET PARMIGIANO:** Add ¼ cup Walnut Parmesan (page 230) when adding the fried onions.

**ROSEMARY AND GARLIC CARROTS AND PARSNIPS:** Replace the turnips and beets with carrots and parsnips, peeled and cut into 1-inch pieces. Omit the black pepper. Toss the carrots and parsnips with the oil and salt, plus 1 teaspoon garlic powder and 1 teaspoon dried rosemary.

**TIP:** *For even cooking, the vegetables should be spread out in one layer. If they don't all fit in one layer on the baking sheet, use 2 baking sheets.*

# Baked Fries and Gravy

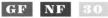

**GF** **NF** 30

Nonstick cooking spray

2 large russet potatoes,
   cut into wedges

Sea salt

Freshly ground black pepper

Old Bay seasoning (optional)

Garlic powder (optional)

Mushroom Gravy (page 228)

SERVES 2 • PREP TIME: 10 MINUTES • COOK TIME: 25 MINUTES

Tony's Diner was one of my favorite hangouts as a teenager in Saginaw, Michigan. My friends and I would meet there and discuss the game plan for the day. Family functions were held there, and it was just across the street from my middle school, making skipping class a necessity at times. Fries and gravy were a staple at Tony's, and this recipe takes me right back.

**1.** Preheat the oven to 475°F. Line a baking sheet with parchment paper, and lightly coat it with nonstick cooking spray.

**2.** Spread out the potato wedges on the prepared baking sheet and spray them lightly. Sprinkle with whichever seasonings you are using, and toss to coat.

**3.** Bake for 10 minutes, flip with a spatula, add additional seasoning if desired, and bake for an additional 5 to 10 minutes, until fork–tender.

**4.** Transfer to a serving plate and top with as much Mushroom Gravy as you like.

### VARIATIONS

**CHILI CHEESE FRIES:** Instead of gravy, top the fries with Slow-Cooker Black Bean Taco Chili (page 50) and Easy Cheese Sauce (page 224).

**DISCO FRIES:** Slather these baked bites in both gravy and Easy Cheese Sauce (page 224). Garnish with some thinly sliced scallions and serve 'em up piping hot.

**TIP:** *Cut your potato wedges in similar sizes so they cook evenly. You can get about 16 wedges out of one large potato.*

# Sweet Potato Mac

1¾ cups water

1 medium sweet potato, peeled and cut into 1-inch cubes

1 carrot, peeled and cut into 1-inch pieces

1 tablespoon plus ¼ cup olive oil, divided

½ onion, chopped

½ cup chopped red bell pepper

3 garlic cloves, minced

Juice of ½ lime

1 tablespoon Dijon mustard

1 teaspoon sea salt

1 pound elbow macaroni, cooked

**SERVES 8 TO 10 • PREP TIME: 10 MINUTES • COOK TIME: 15 MINUTES**

This recipe is more of a delicious macaroni with a creamy sauce. If you want the "cheese" version, simply head to that variation. Another route is to make some Easy Cheese Sauce (page 224) and mix that up with some pasta. I do it all the time and it's divine. But if you are looking for a no-muss, no-fuss start that requires ingredients that you will absolutely find in any standard supermarket, this recipe does the trick.

**1.** Pour the water into a large saucepot and add the sweet potato and carrot. Cover and bring to a boil over medium-high heat. Cook for 10 minutes, or until the vegetables are fork-tender: soft but not falling apart. Remove the pot from the heat but *do not drain the water*.

**2.** In a medium skillet, heat 1 tablespoon of olive oil over medium heat, add the onion and bell pepper and sauté for 3 minutes, or until soft. Add the garlic and sauté for 1 additional minute, or until fragrant.

**3.** Transfer the contents of the saucepot (including the water) to a blender, along with the contents of the skillet. Add the remaining ¼ cup of olive oil, lime juice, mustard, and salt. Blend, starting on the lowest speed and increasing gradually, for 2 minutes, or until smooth and creamy. If you have an immersion blender, add the skillet contents to the saucepot and blend.

**4.** Toss with the cooked pasta.

## VARIATIONS

**HAMBURGER HELPER:** Mix in vegan beef crumbles for a trip down memory lane.

**MAC AND CHEESE:** Here it is, the obligatory macaroni and cheese recipe: Add ¼ cup water, ¼ cup nutritional yeast, and 1 tablespoon white miso paste to the blender. Blend until smooth. Taste the sauce and add up to 1 additional tablespoon of miso, if desired.

**TIP:** *Heat and blenders don't mix. Be sure to remove the center plug from the lid of the blender to release the steam, or else you will have an explosion. Hold a towel firmly over the hole in the lid while blending to avoid a mess.*

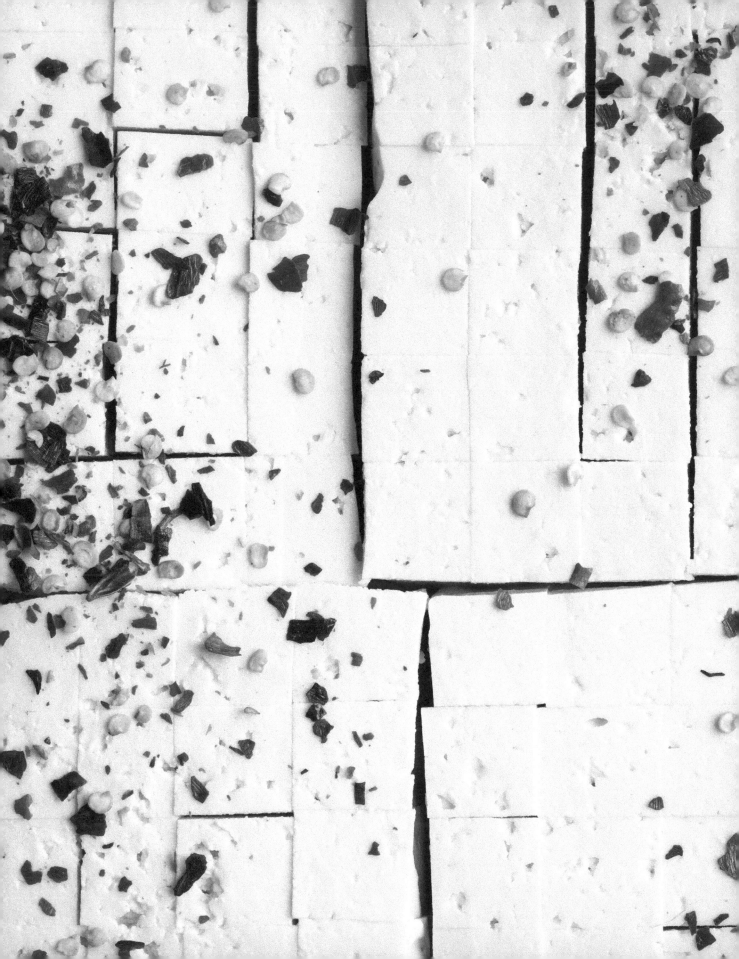

# CHAPTER 8
# Tofu

There are a lot of meat alternatives on the market, but I decided to use only tofu in this chapter because that has been the easiest meat alternative to find for as long as I can remember.

There's also seitan and tempeh. Seitan, sometimes called "wheat meat," is made of vital wheat gluten. It is full of gluten glory and can be used in a multitude of ways to create a meaty supplement for dishes. Tempeh is a traditional soy product (although there are now soy-free versions) made by a controlled fermentation process that binds the soy together into a cake-like form. You can find both seitan and tempeh packaged in different flavors and variations at many health food stores, and even some grocery stores these days. Swap out the tofu in any of these recipes for seitan or tempeh, though I suggest starting with tofu and exploring from there.

In the last few years we have been blessed to have companies that are producing tasty vegan chicken, beef, and pork. By all means, if you find a brand you love, use it in place of the tofu in any of these recipes. But tofu is beautiful because it takes on the flavors you create, making it extremely versatile.

# Basic Baked Tofu

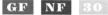 GF NF 30

1 (14-ounce) block extra-firm tofu,
drained and cut into 1-inch cubes

SERVES 4 • PREP TIME: 5 MINUTES • COOK TIME: 20 MINUTES

I have always pressed tofu before cooking it. For this book I wanted to create a method that would speed things up and skip the pressing part, to stick with our theme—*simple*. I believe I found the answer. Baking the tofu like this makes the outside slightly crisp while keeping the inside light and fluffy, making it the perfect vehicle for several recipes in this book.

**1.** Preheat the oven to 425°F. Line a baking sheet with parchment paper.

**2.** Spread the tofu cubes evenly on the prepared baking sheet. Bake for 10 minutes, flip with a spatula, and bake for an additional 10 minutes, or until lightly golden.

**TIP:** *I'm including the basic method here, as well as within the procedures in this chapter; turn to this page when you need a resource for the recipes that are not in this chapter— although this method is so simple that you will be doing it from memory after just a few times.*

# Scrappy Scrambler

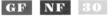

1 (14-ounce) block extra-firm
   tofu, drained

2 tablespoons vegan butter, melted

¼ cup low-sodium vegetable broth

1¼ teaspoons sea salt, plus more
   if needed

1 teaspoon garlic powder

½ teaspoon ground turmeric

½ teaspoon black pepper, plus more
   if needed

1 tablespoon olive oil

½ cup diced onion

½ cup diced red bell pepper

1 cup stemmed and sliced baby bella
   or white button mushrooms

1 (5-ounce) package baby spinach

2 scallions, thinly sliced, for garnish

**SERVES 4 • PREP TIME: 10 MINUTES • COOK TIME: 15 MINUTES**

Tofu scrambles get a bad rep sometimes, and I can understand why. I often find them to be too dry or lacking in flavor. But that all changes with this recipe. I serve it up to friends and family with pride, and I hope you will, too.

**1.** Cut the tofu into 4 equal sections. Crumble one section into a blender. Set the rest aside.

**2.** Add the butter, broth, salt, garlic powder, turmeric, and pepper to the blender and blend until smooth.

**3.** Heat the oil in a medium skillet over medium-high heat. Add the onion, bell pepper, and mushrooms and sauté for 3 to 5 minutes, until soft. Crumble the remaining tofu into the skillet and mix well to combine. Sauté for 2 minutes. Add the blended-tofu mixture and toss to coat the scramble completely. Add the spinach and stir it in until wilted, about 3 minutes.

**4.** Let the mixture simmer for 5 minutes to cook the liquid down a bit, stirring occasionally. Season with more salt and pepper, if desired. Garnish with the scallions.

### VARIATIONS

**DELUXE SAUSAGE SCRAMBLE:** Add your favorite vegan sausage, crumbled or chopped, along with chopped tomato and vegan cheddar shreds.

**BREAKFAST BURRITO:** Divide this mixture among three 10-inch burrito tortillas, drizzle with Garlic-Sriracha Aioli (page 223), and roll 'em up.

**TIP:** *If you can get your hands on Himalayan black salt (kala namak), add ¾ teaspoon to the blended tofu mixture to take your scramble to the next level. The sulfur in the salt will make anyone think they are actually eating eggs.*

# Mini Tofu Quiche

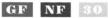

Nonstick cooking spray

1 (14-ounce) block extra-firm tofu, drained

½ cup low-sodium vegetable broth

2 tablespoons olive oil

1 tablespoon cornstarch

1 teaspoon onion powder

1 teaspoon garlic powder

½ teaspoon ground turmeric

1 teaspoon sea salt

½ cup chopped onion

½ red bell pepper, chopped

1 cup stemmed and diced baby bellas or white button mushrooms

1 teaspoon dried rosemary

**SERVES 6 · PREP TIME: 10 MINUTES · COOK TIME: 20 MINUTES**

Quiche isn't just for breakfast anymore. This is a great make-ahead recipe to have as a snack or to take with you to work for lunch. Once you get comfortable with the recipe, I highly encourage you to start playing around in the kitchen, mixing in your favorite veggies.

**1.** Preheat the oven to 425°F. Lightly coat a 12-cup muffin tin with nonstick cooking spray.

**2.** In a blender, blend the tofu, broth, oil, cornstarch, onion powder, garlic powder, turmeric, and salt until smooth and creamy. Transfer to a large bowl.

**3.** Add the onion, bell pepper, mushrooms, and rosemary to the tofu mixture. Mix until well combined.

**4.** Drop ¼ cup of the tofu mixture into each greased muffin cup. Bake for 20 to 25 minutes, until a toothpick inserted in the middle of a quiche comes out clean.

## VARIATIONS

**SAUSAGE AND CHEDDAR QUICHE:** Omit the onion, bell pepper, mushrooms, and rosemary. Instead, add 2 vegan sausage links, chopped or crumbled, along with ¾ cup vegan cheese shreds to the tofu mixture.

**FETA AND SUN-DRIED TOMATO QUICHE:** Omit the onion, bell pepper, and rosemary. Add ¾ cup crumbled Fast Feta (page 225) and ½ cup chopped sun-dried tomatoes to the tofu mixture, along with the mushrooms.

**TIP:** *If you have picky eaters and want the vegetables softer, sauté them in a skillet in 1 tablespoon olive oil for 3 to 5 minutes before adding them to the tofu mixture.*

# Tofu Benedict Florentine

1 (14-ounce) block extra-firm
  tofu, drained

1 teaspoon olive oil

1 (10-ounce) package baby spinach

1 cup Mayonnaise (page 223) or
  store-bought vegan mayonnaise

3 tablespoons vegan butter, melted

1 teaspoon lemon juice

1 teaspoon hot sauce

½ teaspoon ground turmeric

¼ teaspoon black pepper

4 vegan English muffins, toasted

Chopped fresh parsley, for garnish
  (optional)

**SERVES 4 · PREP TIME: 5 MINUTES · COOK TIME: 25 MINUTES**

As delicious as eggs Benedict were to me back in the day, I couldn't help but think, "This is everything I should not be eating for breakfast" each time I decided to indulge. Now all that has changed with the elimination of the eggs and bacon, and the addition of a dose of greens and protein to take their place. While it still isn't exactly health food, I don't feel as guilty with this version. If you've picked up some Himalayan black salt (kala namak), this is another recipe it works well with, although it's not required. Just sprinkle some on after the tofu is baked—a little goes a long way.

1. Preheat the oven to 425°F. Line a baking sheet with parchment paper.

2. Slice the tofu horizontally into 4 thin sheets, then cut each sheet crosswise into 4 pieces, for a total of 16 pieces. Spread the tofu in a single layer on the prepared baking sheet and bake for 10 minutes. Flip and bake for an additional 10 minutes, or until lightly crisped on both sides.

3. Meanwhile, heat the oil in a large skillet over medium heat. Add the spinach and toss with a spatula or tongs frequently for 2 minutes, or until wilted down. You may have to cook the spinach in two batches, adding another teaspoon of oil if needed.

4. In a small saucepot, combine the mayonnaise, butter, lemon juice, hot sauce, turmeric, and pepper. Stir over medium-low heat until just warmed.

5. Serve open-faced with each side of a toasted English muffin topped with some spinach, 2 tofu pieces, and the sauce spooned over the top. Garnish with parsley, if desired.

**VARIATIONS**

**BASIC BENEDICT:** Omit the spinach. Sear vegan ham deli slices, Portobello Bacon (page 185), or the thinly sliced vegan protein of your choice in 1 teaspoon oil in a skillet until slightly browned and crisp. Layer the ham between the English muffin and the tofu. Top with the sauce.

**BENEDICT BURGERS:** Place Southwest Pinto Bean Burger (page 56) patties between toasted vegan hamburger buns and add the baked tofu and sauce.

**TIP:** *Don't get discouraged when looking for vegan English muffins at the store. You will find several brands that are not vegan, but I promise you they exist. Who knows, maybe it's the brand you are currently enjoying!*

# Buffalo Tofu Sandwich Roll with Ranch Dressing

30

1 (14-ounce) block extra-firm tofu, drained

1 cup hot sauce (Frank's RedHot preferred)

2 tablespoons vegan butter

1 tablespoon dark-brown sugar

½ teaspoon garlic powder

½ teaspoon onion powder

½ teaspoon sea salt

6 romaine lettuce leaves, shredded

6 vegan hot dog buns, toasted

Unhidden Valley Ranch Dressing (page 221) or store-bought vegan ranch dressing

2 scallions, thinly sliced

**SERVES 6 • PREP TIME: 5 MINUTES • COOK TIME: 20 MINUTES**

The best Buffalo sandwich I ever had came from a lovely place in Fort Lauderdale, Florida, called Green Bar and Kitchen. This place is owned by some of the nicest people, Charlie and Elena. You can see more about them and their restaurant in *The Vegan Roadie* Fort Lauderdale episode. I was obsessed with their buffalo tempeh sandwich and wanted to come up with a super-simple version I could toss together for lunch. This is it, and I hope you love it as much as I do.

**1.** Preheat the oven to 425°F. Line a baking sheet with parchment paper.

**2.** Cut the tofu horizontally into 2 thin sheets, then cut each sheet crosswise into 6 pieces, for a total of 12 pieces. Spread them out on the baking sheet and bake for 10 minutes, flip with a spatula, and bake for an additional 10 minutes, or until lightly golden.

**3.** Meanwhile, in a medium saucepan, mix together the hot sauce, butter, sugar, garlic powder, onion powder, and salt. Bring just to a boil over medium heat, then reduce to a simmer and cook until the butter is completely melted and the sugar has dissolved. Remove from the heat.

**4.** When the tofu is done baking, drizzle half of the Buffalo sauce over the tofu on the baking sheet and toss gently with a spatula until coated.

**5.** Build each sandwich by placing some shredded romaine on one side of the bun and 2 tofu pieces on the other side. Drizzle the tofu first with the remaining Buffalo sauce and then with some ranch, and finish off with a scattering of scallions.

## VARIATIONS

**BUFFALO TOFU SALAD:** Chop up a head of romaine lettuce, add some shredded carrot and chopped celery, and top with the Buffalo tofu and Unhidden Valley Ranch Dressing (page 221).

**BUFFALO TEMPEH SANDWICH ROLL:** Instead of the tofu, use 1 (8-ounce) package tempeh, steamed over a low heat and cut into planks, for a heartier texture. Double the sauce ingredients in a skillet and cook the tempeh in the sauce, covered, for 20 minutes, or until the liquid has reduced and the tempeh is well coated. Then build the sandwiches as specified.

**TIP:** *I toast my bun on an open flame, laying the bun halves face down on the grate of my stovetop. This method gives the bread a rustic look and taste, but you have to be careful it doesn't burn. I use tongs to manage the bun from a safe distance.*

# BBQ Hawaiian Tofu Bowl

 **NF** 30

SERVES 4 · PREP TIME: 10 MINUTES · COOK TIME: 20 MINUTES

1 large red onion, cut into ¼-inch slices

1 red bell pepper, seeded and cut into ¼-inch slices

1 tablespoon plus 1 teaspoon olive oil, plus more as needed, divided

1 (14-ounce) block extra-firm tofu, drained and cut into 1-inch cubes

1 (20-ounce) can sliced pineapple, drained, or 1 pineapple, peeled, cored, and cut into ¼-inch slices

1 cup Basic BBQ Sauce (page 232) or store-bought barbecue sauce

1 (5-ounce) package baby spinach

1 cup cooked quinoa

Chopped fresh cilantro, for garnish (optional)

A serving of greens, pineapple, and protein balance this sweet and savory bowl perfectly. It does get a little involved, with a pan in the oven and a skillet on the stovetop, but it's straightforward. I won't be mad at you for picking up barbecue sauce at the store to cut down on steps; keep it as simple as you need.

**1.** Preheat the oven to 425°F. Line a large baking sheet with parchment paper.

**2.** In a bowl, toss the onion and bell pepper with 1 tablespoon of olive oil. Spread them out on half of the prepared baking sheet. Spread out the tofu cubes on the other half. Bake for 10 minutes, toss with a spatula, and bake for 10 more minutes.

**3.** While the tofu and vegetables are baking, heat the remaining 1 teaspoon of olive oil in a large skillet over medium-high heat. Add the pineapple slices in batches and sauté until darkly browned on both sides, adding more oil as needed.

**4.** Toss the baked tofu with the barbecue sauce until thoroughly coated.

**5.** Divide the spinach and quinoa among 4 bowls. Top with the vegetables, tofu, and pineapple. Garnish with cilantro, if desired. →

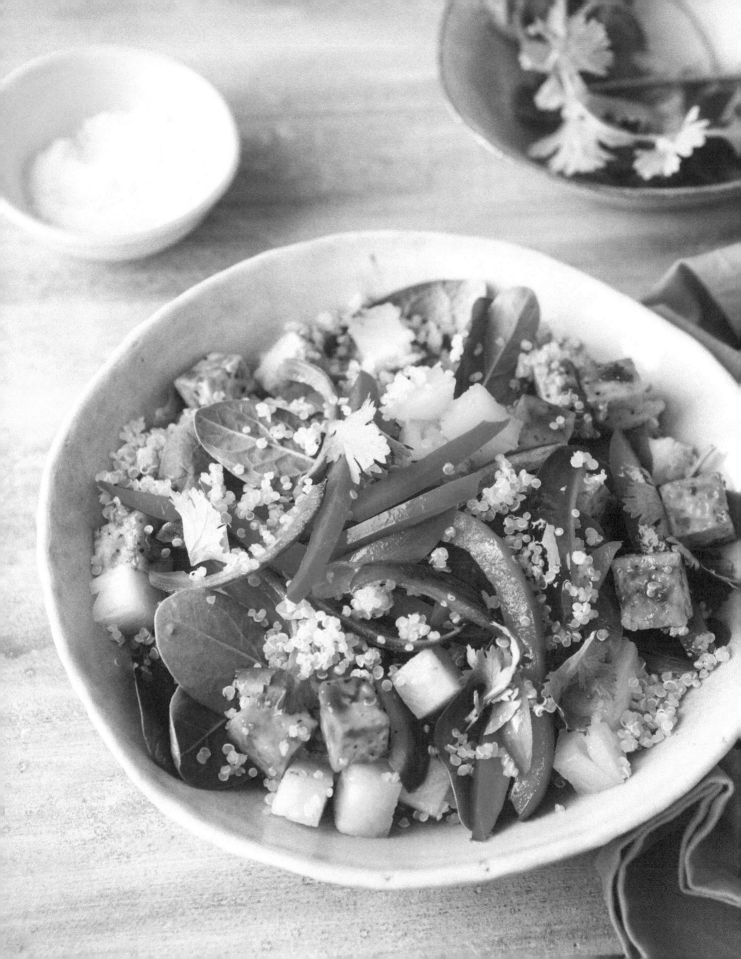

### VARIATIONS

**MEDITERRANEAN SPINACH BOWL:** Replace the red onion with 1 (14-ounce) can quartered artichokes, drained and roughly chopped, and bake with the bell pepper and tofu as directed. Divide the baked tofu, bell pepper, and artichokes among 4 bowls filled with spinach and quinoa. Omit the pineapple and barbecue sauce. Drizzle each bowl with 1 teaspoon olive oil and a squeeze of lemon juice. Dollop 2 tablespoons White Bean Hummus (page 43) in the center of each bowl. Garnish with 1 tablespoon sliced green olives.

**SWEET-AND-SOUR CAULIFLOWER BOWL:** Omit the tofu. Replace the red bell pepper with a green bell pepper and bake with the onion as directed. Divide the bell pepper and onion among 4 bowls filled with spinach and quinoa. Omit the pineapple and barbecue sauce. Top each bowl with Roasted Sweet-and-Sour Cauliflower (page 116). Sprinkle with white sesame seeds, if desired.

**TIP:** *Sprinkle the bowl with chopped almonds, chia seeds, or hemp seeds for an extra serving of protein.*

# Chicken-Free Tofu and Apple Salad

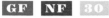

1 (14-ounce) block extra-firm tofu, drained, pressed (see Tip), and cut into ½-inch cubes

2 cups chopped apple (preferably Red Delicious, Braeburn, or Fuji)

¼ cup minced onion

¼ cup thinly sliced celery

1 tablespoon chopped fresh parsley

¾ teaspoon dried dill

½ teaspoon garlic powder

½ teaspoon onion powder

½ cup Mayonnaise (page 223) or store-bought vegan mayonnaise

½ teaspoon sea salt, plus more if needed

½ teaspoon black pepper, plus more if needed

I was always skeptical about eating chicken or tuna salad—until I went vegan. Funny how the brain works! The minute I started exploring how to veganize these popular mayonnaise-based salads, I was delighted at how easily they came together and how versatile they are. This recipe is great on salads, sandwiches, or wraps.

**1.** In a large bowl, toss together the tofu cubes, apple, onion, celery, parsley, dill, garlic powder, and onion powder until well combined.

**2.** Fold in the mayonnaise and add the salt and pepper. Adjust the salt and pepper to taste.

### VARIATIONS

**MEDITERRANEAN CHICKEN-FREE SALAD:** Omit the apple and onion. Add ¼ cup minced red onion and ½ cup pitted and chopped green or kalamata olives.

**WALDORF CHICKEN-FREE SALAD:** Omit the apple and onion. Add ¼ cup chopped walnuts and 2 cups halved grapes.

**TIP:** *Pressing tofu eliminates extra water content, so you aren't left with a soupy salad. To press it without a tofu press, drain the tofu and wrap generously in paper towels. Set the tofu in a large, shallow bowl and place a saucepot or skillet on top of it with something heavy inside, like a couple of canned items or a bag of flour or sugar. Let it sit for about 25 minutes, until the tofu is drier. Discard the liquid you squeezed out.*

# Tofu Pesto Bowl

**GF** **30**

1 (14-ounce) block extra-firm tofu, drained and cut into 1-inch cubes

1 tablespoon olive oil

½ cup sliced onion

1 bunch curly kale, stemmed and roughly chopped

Sea salt

Black pepper

1 cup Pistachio Pesto (page 226) or store-bought vegan pesto

2 cups cooked brown rice

**TIP:** *A spiralizer is a fun tool to have on hand to create healthy meals that look like a food we all love, pasta. You may be able to find a spiralizer in the kitchenware area at your grocery store, but if not, just order one online; they are inexpensive. A potato peeler also does the trick for creating wide, flat noodles, if you're just dabbling in vegetable pasta–bilities.*

SERVES 4 • PREP TIME: 10 MINUTES • COOK TIME: 20 MINUTES

I have this beautiful friend, Meghan, who shines light everywhere she goes. She's that person everyone wants to know the instant they meet her. But two things make her light up beyond her normal brightness: pesto and soy milk creamer. To say she is a pesto aficionado is putting it mildly. This entire dish has been Meghan-approved with shining colors. Perhaps you will light up with joy just as she does when you take your first bite.

**1.** Preheat the oven to 425°F. Line a baking sheet with parchment paper.

**2.** Spread the tofu cubes in a single layer on the prepared baking sheet and bake for 10 minutes. Flip with a spatula and bake for an additional 10 minutes, or until lightly browned.

**3.** Heat the oil in a large skillet over medium heat. Add the onion and sauté for 3 minutes, or until soft and stringy. Add the kale and sauté for about 3 minutes more, tossing frequently, until wilted. Season with salt and pepper.

**4.** In a large bowl, toss the baked tofu with the pesto.

**5.** Divide the rice among 4 bowls and top with the kale mixture and pesto tofu.

### VARIATIONS

**GARDEN VEGETABLE TOFU PESTO BOWL:** After sautéing the onion, add another 1 tablespoon olive oil, ½ cup corn kernels, ½ cup halved cherry tomatoes, and ½ cup thinly sliced zucchini to the skillet. Cook for 3 to 5 minutes, until soft. Season with salt and pepper, add the kale, and continue as directed.

**RAW NOODLES AND PESTO TOFU:** Omit the onion, kale, and rice. With a potato peeler or spiralizer, create a bowl full of raw "noodles" with carrots, zucchini, and yellow squash. Top with the tofu pesto. If you want a little warmth, sauté the noodles in 1 tablespoon olive oil for 3 minutes, or until warmed through.

# Tasty Tofu Pad Thai

**GF** **30**

1 (14-ounce) block extra-firm tofu, drained and cut into 1-inch cubes

½ cup low-sodium vegetable broth

3 tablespoons dark-brown sugar

3 tablespoons creamy peanut butter

2 tablespoons soy sauce or gluten-free tamari

2 tablespoons lime juice

1 to 3 teaspoons sriracha sauce (optional)

4 ounces uncooked rice noodles

2 cups chopped broccoli florets

⅓ cup crushed peanuts, for garnish

2 scallions, thinly sliced, for garnish

Chopped fresh cilantro, for garnish

**TIP:** *For an authentic touch, add tamarind paste to the peanut butter sauce, if you can get your hands on some. Start with ½ teaspoon and add more to your liking.*

SERVES 4 • PREP TIME: 5 MINUTES • COOK TIME: 20 MINUTES

Pad thai shouldn't be complicated—it's all about a decadent and creamy peanut sauce. Aside from crisping up the tofu in the oven, this is a one-pot meal. The most difficult thing to replace in traditional pad thai is the fish sauce, which is what typically rounds out all the flavors. I find the addition of soy sauce and lime juice completes this simple recipe just as nicely.

1. Preheat the oven to 425°F. Line a baking sheet with parchment paper.

2. Spread the tofu cubes on the prepared baking sheet and bake for 10 minutes. Toss with a spatula and bake for 10 additional minutes, or until slightly golden.

3. While the tofu is baking, whisk together the broth, sugar, peanut butter, soy sauce, lime juice, and sriracha (if using) in a small bowl until creamy.

4. Prepare the rice noodles according to the package direction and add the broccoli in the last 2 minutes of boiling. Drain the noodles and broccoli, return to the pot, and toss with the peanut butter sauce and tofu.

5. Divide among 4 bowls and garnish with the crushed peanuts, scallions, and cilantro.

## VARIATIONS

**MUSHROOM PAD THAI:** Omit the tofu. Heat 1 tablespoon toasted sesame oil or olive oil in a large skillet over medium heat and add 2 (8-ounce) packages baby bella or white button mushrooms, stemmed and sliced. Sauté the mushrooms for 5 minutes, or until they're reduced in size. Mix in the mushrooms instead of the tofu in the recipe.

**VEGGIE DELUXE PAD THAI:** Omit the tofu. Heat 1 tablespoon olive oil in a large skillet over medium heat and add ½ cup julienned carrot, ½ cup stemmed and sliced baby bella or white button mushrooms, ½ cup halved cherry tomatoes, and ½ red bell pepper, diced. Sauté the vegetables for 3 to 5 minutes, until soft. Mix in the vegetables instead of the tofu in the recipe.

# Not Yo Momma's Tofu Piccata

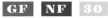

1 (14-ounce) block extra-firm tofu, drained

1 tablespoon olive oil

1 onion, chopped

3 garlic cloves, minced

¼ teaspoon sea salt

¼ teaspoon black pepper

1¼ cups low-sodium vegetable broth, divided

1 tablespoon cornstarch

Juice of 1½ lemons

2 tablespoons vegan butter

2 tablespoons capers, drained

3 tablespoons chopped fresh parsley, divided

SERVES 4 • PREP TIME: 10 MINUTES • COOK TIME: 20 MINUTES

A long, long time ago, I spent a summer waiting tables at the Cheesecake Factory in Seattle. I was in my mid-twenties and able to eat anything and everything I wanted without it wreaking havoc on my digestive system or waistline . . . ah, youth. I remember huge plates of chicken piccata that I would eat in one sitting on my 30-minute break. Behavior like that would be disastrous now. Thankfully, I've created a more compassionate, healthful, and portion-conscious version for us all to enjoy.

1. Preheat the oven to 425°F. Line a baking sheet with parchment paper.

2. Cut the tofu horizontally into 3 thin sheets, then cut each sheet in half crosswise. Cut the resulting 6 pieces on a diagonal to create a total of 12 triangles. Place the triangles on the prepared baking sheet and bake for 10 minutes. Flip with a spatula and bake for an additional 10 minutes.

3. While the tofu is baking, heat the oil in a large skillet over medium heat. Sauté the onion for 3 minutes, or until soft. Add the garlic and sauté for 1 additional minute, or until fragrant.

4. Add the salt, pepper, and 1 cup of broth to the skillet; add the broth slowly to avoid spattering. Reduce the heat to a simmer.

5. In a small bowl, whisk the cornstarch into the remaining ¼ cup of broth to create a slurry. Slowly pour the slurry into the skillet, stirring until the sauce begins to thicken.

6. Add the lemon juice, butter, capers, and 2 tablespoons of parsley. Mix until the butter is melted and the ingredients are well combined.

7. Dredge the tofu through the piccata sauce to fully coat, and transfer to a serving plate. Drizzle generously with the remaining sauce. Garnish with the remaining 1 tablespoon of parsley.

**VARIATIONS**

**TEMPEH PICCATA:** Cut 1 (8-ounce) package tempeh into 12 triangles as directed for the tofu. Steam the tempeh triangles for 20 minutes, then pan-fry them in a skillet in olive oil. Make the sauce in a different skillet.

**QUICK TOFU PARMIGIANO:** Slice and bake the tofu as directed. Instead of the piccata sauce, serve the tofu atop cooked pasta, topped with Magnificent Marinara (page 231), Easy Cheese Sauce–Mozzarella variation (page 224), and Walnut Parmesan (page 230). If you prefer to use store-bought vegan mozzarella shreds, pop the dressed tofu under the broiler for 3 to 5 minutes to melt the cheese. Sprinkle with chopped fresh basil.

**TIP:** *Tempeh is one of my absolute favorite protein alternatives. It's heartier than tofu and offers a different texture entirely. If your supermarket carries it, I highly recommend you swap it out in some of these tofu recipes after you get comfortable with them. Just be sure to steam it for 20 minutes first, as it will be slightly bitter if you don't.*

# Tofu Marsala

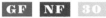 

1 (14-ounce) block extra-firm tofu, drained

1 tablespoon olive oil

1 onion, chopped

3 garlic cloves, minced

½ cup dry Marsala wine or Marsala cooking wine

2 (8-ounce) packages baby bella or white button mushrooms, stemmed and sliced

1 cup low-sodium vegetable broth

1 tablespoon tomato paste

1 tablespoon cornstarch

Sea salt

Black pepper

Chopped fresh parsley, for garnish

**SERVES 4 · PREP TIME: 10 MINUTES · COOK TIME: 20 MINUTES**

Marsala is Italian-American food, a variation of the traditional Italian scaloppine dishes. Contrary to popular belief, food in Italy is more often than not created with a base of grains, greens, and beans. You can learn more about vegan food in Italy by watching Season 3 of *The Vegan Roadie: Ciao Italia!* For now, whip up this recipe and serve it with some greens for a healthful, satisfying meal.

**1.** Preheat the oven to 425°F. Line a baking sheet with parchment paper.

**2.** Cut the tofu horizontally into 3 thin sheets, then cut each sheet in half crosswise. Cut the resulting 6 pieces on a diagonal to create a total of 12 triangles. Place the triangles on the prepared baking sheet and bake for 10 minutes. Flip with a spatula and bake for an additional 10 minutes.

**3.** While the tofu is baking, heat the oil in a large skillet over medium heat. Add the onion and sauté for 3 minutes, or until soft. Add the garlic and sauté for 1 additional minute, or until fragrant.

**4.** Add the wine and mushrooms to the skillet. Cook for 5 to 7 minutes, until the wine has reduced and the mushrooms have reduced in size.

**5.** In a small bowl, whisk together the broth, tomato paste, and cornstarch to make a thick slurry. Drizzle the slurry slowly into the skillet and stir until thickened, about 3 minutes. Season with salt and pepper.

**6.** Dredge the tofu through the sauce in the skillet to coat, then transfer to a serving plate. Drizzle generously with the remaining wine-mushroom mixture. Garnish with parsley.

## VARIATIONS

**MEDITERRANEAN MARSALA:** Replace 1 cup of the mushrooms with 1 cup roughly chopped canned and drained artichokes.

**STUFFED MARSALA TOFU:** Create layers with a piece of baked tofu, followed by some Warm Lentil Salad (page 69), topped with another piece of baked tofu, and drizzled with the Marsala sauce. Use toothpicks if there is an issue keeping the top layer of tofu in place.

**TIP:** *I would typically use shallots in this recipe, but I went for an onion to maintain the "simple" factor. If you are feeling adventurous, grab 3 shallots and use them in place of the onion here. They create a sweeter, milder flavor, with less of a bite than an onion, but also have a hint of a garlic taste for a perfect balance.*

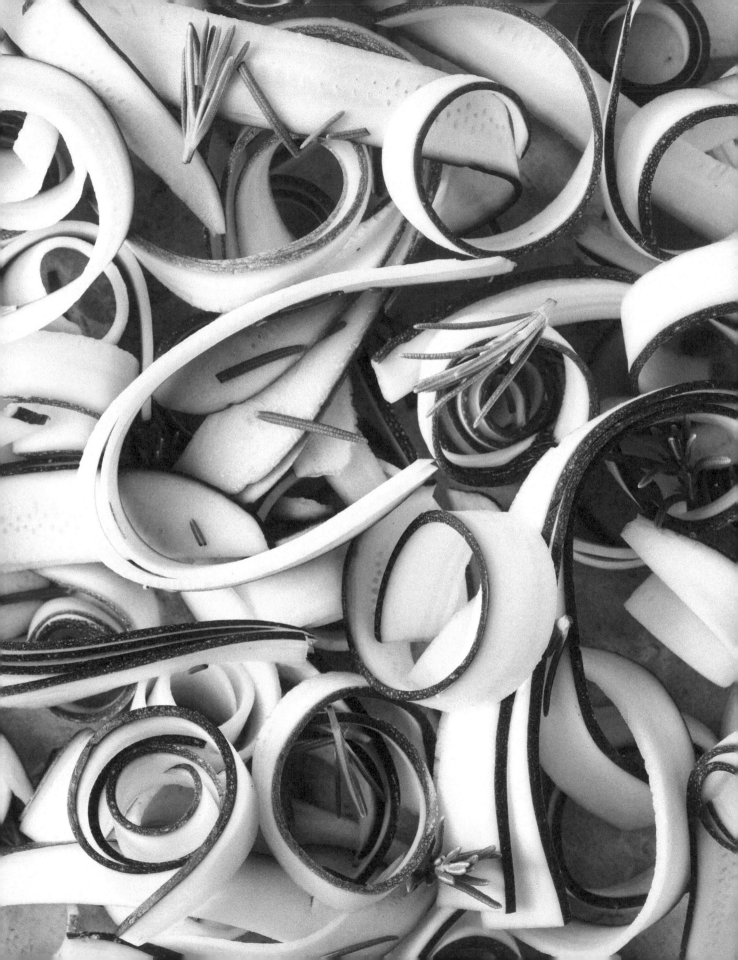

# CHAPTER 9
# Squash

Hold on to your hat, Aunt Ethel, squash is actually a fruit. Yes, ma'am. But in the culinary world we use them as vegetables. I suppose this makes sense because the many varieties of squash just aren't made to be enjoyed as one would an apple or a peach; they're better cooked. Summer squash (the soft ones, like zucchini) and winter squash (the hard ones, like butternut) require different cooking techniques and preparation, but both are extremely versatile.

From making noodles and bread to grilling with just a little oil on a summer day, the options for zucchini are endless. As a good friend of mine said, "I love zucchini—they taste like summer." She couldn't be more right, as their peak season is June through August. So snag those bad boys when they are vibrant and full of color and flavor.

Winter squashes are fun and unique. While some may be a little hard to find, like lakota, arikara, and turban squash, you can find acorn, butternut, kabocha, and spaghetti squash in just about every supermarket. They are the types we will focus on in this chapter. As you start to play with these recipes and become more comfortable with the ingredients, I encourage you to up your squash game and bring home some of the more unusual offerings. There is a world of discovery out there when it comes to the gourd family.

# Creamy Butternut Squash Soup

**GF** **NF** **SF** 30

1 butternut squash (roughly 2 pounds), peeled, seeded, and cut into ½-inch cubes

1 red bell pepper, seeded and chopped

1 large onion, chopped

3 garlic cloves, minced

4 cups low-sodium vegetable broth

Juice of ½ lemon

2 tablespoons maple syrup

¾ teaspoon salt

¾ teaspoon black pepper

**TIP:** *Make this ahead and heat as needed throughout the week. It will keep for up to a week in the refrigerator or up to a month in the freezer.*

SERVES 4 TO 6 • PREP TIME: 10 MINUTES • COOK TIME: 20 MINUTES

No need for heavy cream to achieve a decadent and rich texture in your soup—just let the veggies and a blender handle the task. Soup has always been helpful when I'm trying to maintain my weight, but the canned ones are full of sodium. Keep this recipe on hand for a quick, guilt-free, and satisfying lunch or dinner.

**1.** In a large stockpot, combine the squash, bell pepper, onion, garlic, and broth. Mix well to combine, cover, and bring to a boil. Reduce to a simmer and cook, covered, for 15 minutes, or until the squash is fork-tender. Add the lemon juice, maple syrup, salt, and pepper and stir well to combine.

**2.** Carefully transfer the soup to a blender. Remove the plug from the blender lid to allow steam to escape, hold a towel firmly over the hole in the lid, and blend until smooth. Start on the lowest speed possible and increase gradually until the soup is completely smooth. Depending on your blender capacity, this might have to be done in two batches. (If you have an immersion blender, it would work great here.)

**3.** Gently reheat over a low heat to serve.

## VARIATIONS

**BUTTERNUT PASTA FAGIOLI:** After the soup is completely blended and creamy, return it to the stockpot and add 1 (14-ounce) can diced tomatoes with their juice; 1 (14-ounce) can cannellini beans, rinsed and drained; and ½ pound elbow macaroni or small shells, cooked. Stir well to combine and let sit for 3 minutes to warm through.

**BUTTERNUT SQUASH WITH ITALIAN SAUSAGE AND CORN:** After the soup is completely blended and creamy, return it to the stockpot. In a medium skillet, heat 1 tablespoon olive oil over medium heat. Add 1 cup corn kernels and sauté for 4 to 6 minutes, until they're starting to brown. Add 2 vegan Italian sausages, cut into ¼-inch-thick slices, and sauté for an additional 2 to 4 minutes, until crispy. Mix the sausage and corn into the soup until well combined.

# Red Curry Kabocha Squash

   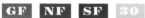

SERVES 4 • PREP TIME: 15 MINUTES • COOK TIME: 15 MINUTES

1 tablespoon olive oil

1 onion, chopped

1 green bell pepper, seeded and chopped

1 kabocha squash (about 1½ pounds), peeled, seeded, and cut into 1-inch cubes

1 (13.5-ounce) can full-fat coconut milk

4 teaspoons red curry paste, plus more if needed

½ teaspoon sea salt, plus more if needed

Juice of ½ lime

3 tablespoons chopped fresh cilantro, divided

4 cups cooked jasmine rice

**TIP:** *Red curry paste is usually located in the international aisle at the supermarket.*

Most of this chapter is dedicated to squash you may likely already be familiar with, but I wanted to toss in one of my favorites that is common in standard supermarkets but may not be as familiar. The kabocha, a winter squash of the Japanese variety, is a mottled dark green and looks like a flattened sphere. I used it in this curry recipe because the naturally robust, sweet flavors pair nicely with the zesty spices.

**1.** Heat the oil in a large skillet over medium heat. Add the onion and bell pepper and sauté for 5 minutes, or until soft.

**2.** Add the squash, coconut milk, and curry paste and mix until well combined. Bring to a boil, then reduce to a simmer. Cover and cook for 10 minutes, or until the squash is fork-tender. Mix in the salt, lime juice, and 1 tablespoon of cilantro until well combined. Add more salt if desired. You may also add more curry paste at this point if you like more heat.

**3.** Divide the rice among 4 plates and top with the squash mixture. Sprinkle with the remaining 2 tablespoons of cilantro.

### VARIATIONS

**SOUTHWEST KABOCHA SQUASH:** Omit the coconut milk, red curry paste, and jasmine rice. Add 1¼ cups low-sodium vegetable broth and 2 tablespoons Taco Seasoning (page 219) and simmer, covered, for 8 minutes. Add 1 cup frozen or fresh corn kernels and cook for an additional 2 minutes, or until the squash is fork-tender. Use 4 cups of brown rice instead of jasmine rice to serve.

**KABOCHA FRIES:** Preheat the oven to 375°F. Line 2 baking sheets with parchment paper. Leave the skin on the kabocha squash. Cut it in half, seed it, and cut it into ½-inch slices. In a large bowl, toss the kabocha squash slices with 2 tablespoons olive oil and ½ teaspoon sea salt, then spread them evenly on the prepared baking sheet. Bake for 10 minutes, flip, and bake for an additional 5 minutes. Turn the oven to broil and broil for 2 to 4 minutes, until browned. Serve with ketchup or your favorite dipping sauce.

# Maple-Bourbon Acorn Squash

**GF** **NF**

SERVES 4 · PREP TIME: 10 MINUTES · COOK TIME: 30 MINUTES

1 acorn squash (1 to 2 pounds),
    seeded and cut into ½-inch slices

½ cup bourbon

⅓ cup maple syrup

¼ cup vegan butter

¼ teaspoon ground cinnamon

2 pinches sea salt

**TIP:** *You can cook the seeds from any winter squash as you would pumpkin seeds at Halloween. Clean any squash pieces or guts off the seeds and toss with 1 teaspoon olive oil and ¼ teaspoon sea salt. Spread the seeds evenly on a parchment-lined baking sheet and bake at 275°F for 15 minutes, or until just starting to brown. Remove from the oven and let cool before enjoying. These make a great snack.*

Acorn squash is probably my favorite winter squash. Start off with this sweet and boozy version for a quick introduction to its wonders. If you get a chance and you have the time, though, I urge you to also try the Thanksgiving Stuffed Acorn Squash variation. Your dinner guests will thank you.

**1.** Preheat the oven to 425°F. Line a baking sheet with parchment paper.

**2.** Spread the squash slices on the prepared baking sheet and bake for 20 minutes.

**3.** Meanwhile, in a small saucepot, combine the bourbon, maple syrup, and butter. Melt over low heat and stir until well combined.

**4.** Flip the squash, drizzle with the bourbon mixture, and sprinkle with the cinnamon and salt. Bake for 8 to 10 more minutes, until the liquid has started to caramelize and the squash is fork-tender.

## VARIATIONS

**THANKSGIVING STUFFED ACORN SQUASH:** Cut the stem end off 4 acorn squash (the top quarter of each squash) and scoop out the seeds. Cut a coin-size piece off the bottoms so the squashes can stand on their own, then set them upright on a parchment-lined baking sheet. Brush each squash liberally on the insides and the rims with ¼ cup melted vegan butter. Drizzle each with 1 tablespoon maple syrup and sprinkle with paprika. Bake at 375°F for 35 to 45 minutes, until fork-tender, then stuff with warm Stovetop Thanksgiving Rice Stuffing (page 96).

**PROTEIN POWER SQUASH AND QUINOA BOWL:** Top the Rainbow Quinoa Salad (page 92) with Maple-Bourbon Acorn Squash and garnish with pumpkin seeds, chia seeds, and hemp seeds.

# Zucchini Cornbread Muffins

Nonstick cooking spray

1 cup unsweetened soy or almond milk

1 tablespoon apple cider vinegar

1 cup ground yellow cornmeal

¾ cup all-purpose flour

¼ cup organic cane sugar

2 teaspoons baking soda

¾ teaspoon sea salt

¼ cup canola oil

3 cups grated green zucchini

**SERVES 12 • PREP TIME: 10 MINUTES • COOK TIME: 20 MINUTES**

I love zucchini bread because it is so moist and fluffy and delicious. I also love cornbread because it's salty and light. What a sweet partnership these two little lovebirds could have—and now they do. I created these muffins so you can bake them up and take them to a potluck or picnic. Or keep them all for yourself.

**1.** Preheat the oven to 400°F. Lightly coat a 12-cup muffin tin with nonstick cooking spray, or place liners in the muffin tin instead.

**2.** In a small bowl, whisk together the milk and vinegar.

**3.** In a large bowl, whisk together the cornmeal, flour, sugar, baking soda, and salt. Add the milk mixture and canola oil to the dry ingredients and mix until well combined. Fold the zucchini into the batter.

**4.** Fill each muffin cup with ¼ cup batter. Bake for 20 to 22 minutes, until the muffins rise and turn golden on top.

**VARIATIONS**

**JALAPEÑO CORNBREAD MUFFINS:** Omit the zucchini and add 1 minced jalapeño pepper to the batter. Serve with maple butter: ½ cup vegan butter whipped together with 2 tablespoons maple syrup.

**BLUEBERRY CORNBREAD MUFFINS:** Omit the zucchini and add 1½ cups frozen or fresh blueberries instead.

**TIP:** *Grate the zucchini in a food processor with a grater attachment, or use the large holes on a hand or box grater.*

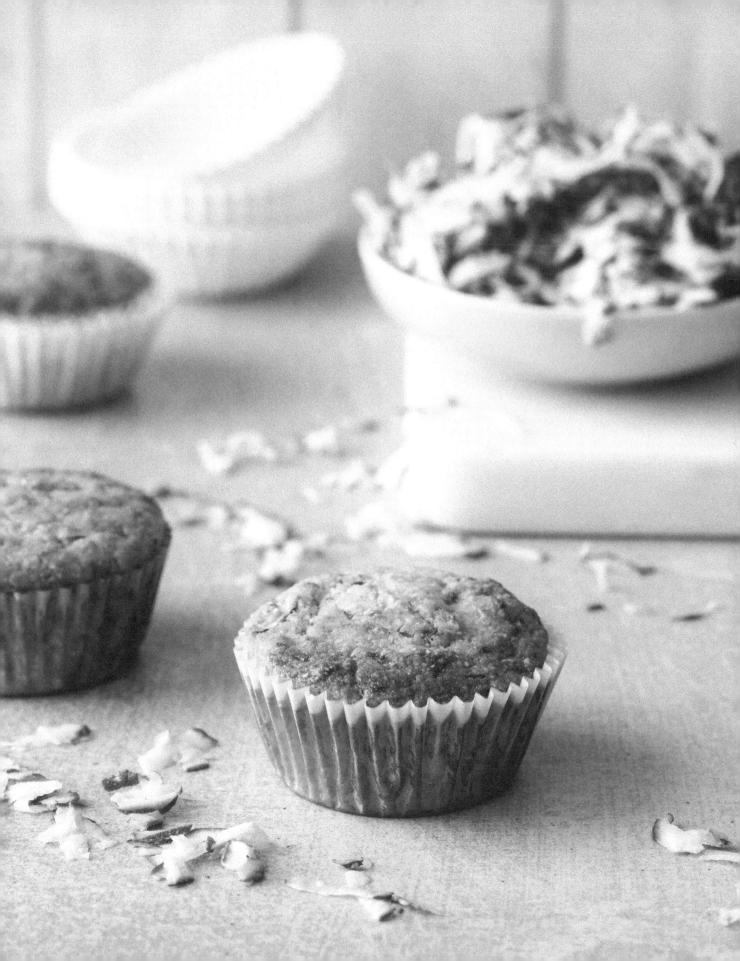

# Buffalo Chickpea Zucchini Boats

2 large green zucchini

1 (15-ounce) can chickpeas, rinsed and drained, half mashed and half left whole

2 cups chopped baby spinach

½ cup hot sauce (Frank's RedHot preferred)

1 tablespoon vegan butter, melted

¼ teaspoon garlic powder

¼ teaspoon onion powder

¼ teaspoon sea salt

Unhidden Valley Ranch Dressing (page 221) or store-bought vegan ranch

Chopped fresh parsley, for garnish

**TIP:** *A melon baller makes the perfect tool for scooping out the insides of summer squash.*

SERVES 4 • PREP TIME: 10 MINUTES • COOK TIME: 20 MINUTES

Zucchini boats are so much fun! This recipe gives you specific measurements, but you will see in the Pizza Zucchini Boats variation that I leave it up to you to get creative. And don't throw away the insides of the zucchini; the Zucchini Toast variation gives you a super-fun and easy option for the tasty flesh.

1. Preheat the oven to 450°F. Line a baking sheet with parchment paper.

2. Cut the zucchini in half lengthwise. Use a spoon to scoop out the insides, leaving at least a ¼-inch-thick wall.

3. In a large bowl, mix together the mashed chickpeas, whole chickpeas, spinach, hot sauce, butter, garlic powder, onion powder, and salt.

4. Transfer the zucchini shells to the prepared baking sheet and fill each with the hot sauce–chickpea mixture.

5. Bake for 15 to 20 minutes, until the zucchini is easily pierced with a fork. Drizzle with ranch dressing and garnish with parsley.

## VARIATIONS

**PIZZA ZUCCHINI BOATS:** Omit everything from the recipe except the hollowed-out zucchini. Add your favorite pizza toppings. I like to use chopped vegan Italian sausage mixed with crumbled Fast Feta (page 225) and Magnificent Marinara (page 231). If you're not using Fast Feta, try 1 (14-ounce) block extra-firm tofu, drained, pressed, and crumbled, to hold it all together. Bake as directed.

**ZUCCHINI TOAST:** Don't let the scooped-out flesh from your zucchini boats go to waste—put it to use on some toast. In a medium skillet, heat 1 tablespoon olive oil. Add ¼ cup minced onion and 2 garlic cloves, minced, and sauté for 1 minute, or until fragrant. Add the zucchini flesh with ¼ teaspoon sea salt and toss to incorporate all the ingredients. Sauté for 5 minutes, or until the zucchini becomes soft. Spread on toast and serve warm.

# Summer Squash Skillet

2 tablespoons olive oil, divided

1 red onion, sliced

3 garlic cloves, sliced

2 medium green zucchini, halved lengthwise and sliced into ¼-inch half moons

2 medium yellow summer squashes, halved lengthwise and sliced into ¼-inch half moons

1 teaspoon Italian seasoning

½ teaspoon sea salt, plus more if needed

¼ teaspoon black pepper, plus more if needed

SERVES 4 TO 6 • PREP TIME: 10 MINUTES •
COOK TIME: 10 MINUTES

This skillet dish is for the summer squash enthusiast. If you have a cast iron skillet, now is the time to put it to use, but any old skillet will do—the largest one you have. If you are lucky enough to have a friend who has a garden and is constantly giving you produce, this recipe will use it up.

**1.** Heat 1 tablespoon of olive oil in a large skillet over medium heat. Add the red onion and sauté for 5 minutes, or until soft and stringy. Add the garlic and sauté for 1 additional minute, or until fragrant.

**2.** Add the remaining 1 tablespoon of olive oil, the zucchini and squashes, Italian seasoning, salt, and pepper. Mix until well combined. Continue cooking for 4 to 6 minutes, tossing the vegetables every couple of minutes to ensure even cooking. The zucchini and yellow squash will start to brown slightly and be fork-tender when ready. Add more salt and pepper to taste.

### VARIATIONS

**SUMMER SQUASH SKILLET FRIED RICE:** Cook everything according to the recipe, then add 3 cups cooked brown rice and 2 tablespoons soy sauce or gluten-free tamari to the skillet. Mix well to combine and cook for an additional 2 to 4 minutes, until everything is heated through. Garnish with chopped scallions.

**VEGGIE VARIETY SUMMER SKILLET:** Omit the yellow squash. Add 1 cup frozen corn kernels, 1 cup whole cherry tomatoes, and 1 cup frozen peas with the zucchini.

**TIP:** *Large zucchini tend to be watery and flavorless, with pulpy insides and large seeds. Try to avoid them, if possible; they should be no longer than 6 to 8 inches. Zucchini with a good amount of the stem still attached will last longer.*

# Slow-Cooker Butternut Squash Risotto

**GF** **NF** **SF**

SERVES 8 TO 10 • PREP TIME: 10 MINUTES • COOK TIME: 3 HOURS

1 butternut squash (roughly
   2 pounds), peeled, seeded,
   and cut into ½-inch cubes

1½ cups uncooked brown rice

1 onion, chopped

4 garlic cloves, minced

1 teaspoon dried thyme

1 teaspoon dried rosemary

4 cups low-sodium vegetable broth

¼ cup Dijon mustard

1 teaspoon sea salt, plus more
   if needed

¼ teaspoon black pepper, plus more
   if needed

**NO SLOW COOKER? NO PROBLEM:**
*To prepare this recipe on the stove,
heat 1 tablespoon olive oil in a
stockpot over medium heat. Add
the onion and garlic and sauté for
2 minutes, or until fragrant. Add the
squash, rice, thyme, rosemary, and
vegetable broth, cover, and simmer
for 40 to 50 minutes. Stir in the
mustard, salt, and pepper. If you find
the mixture still has an excess amount
of liquid, let it simmer, uncovered,
until the liquid evaporates. Keep an
eye on it, and stir occasionally to be
sure the rice doesn't burn.*

This is not a "set it and forget it" while you go to work
slow-cooker recipe, but it is a "set it and forget it" on a
Sunday afternoon while you go to the movies with your
friends and family recipe. Not only that, but it takes
the guesswork and endless stirring out of the typical
approach to risotto. I used brown rice in this recipe,
rather than the Arborio rice that is traditionally used for
risotto, simply because it's healthier. If you choose to use
Arborio rice, the cook time will be less—2 to 2½ hours.

**1.** Combine the squash, rice, onion, garlic, thyme,
rosemary, and broth in a slow cooker, cover, and cook on
high for 3 hours.

**2.** Stir in the mustard, salt, and pepper. Adjust the seasonings to your taste.

## VARIATIONS

**SLOW-COOKER MUSHROOM RISOTTO:** Omit the butternut
squash. Add 2 (8-ounce) packages baby bella or white
button mushrooms, stemmed and quartered.

**SLOW-COOKER CHEESY RISOTTO:** Omit the butternut squash
and Dijon mustard. Cook as directed, and at the end stir
in 1 cup Easy Cheese Sauce (page 224) and ½ cup
Walnut Parmesan (page 230). Garnish with more Walnut
Parmesan and red pepper flakes.

**TIP:** *Slow cookers vary in intensity. If the rice isn't
completely cooked after 3 hours, keep the slow cooker on
the warm setting with the cover on and check back every
15 minutes until the rice has cooked all the way through.*

# Ready-to-Eat Raw Zucchini and Tomato Lasagna

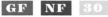  

1 large tomato, sliced ⅛ to
    ¼ inch thick

1 batch Fast Tofu Ricotta (page 225)

1 large green zucchini, peeled,
    halved lengthwise, and sliced into
    ⅛- to ¼-inch half-moons

Balsamic vinegar, for garnish

Chopped fresh basil, for garnish

SERVES 4 • PREP TIME: 10 MINUTES

I love this healthful take on lasagna. The preparation is minimal, so the dish comes together in a matter of minutes for a nourishing dinner or quick lunch. The mixture of tofu and seasonings with a drizzle of balsamic vinegar and some fresh basil give it a decadent quality that always leaves me feeling wealthy in the flavor department.

**1.** Place 1 tomato slice on a serving plate, top with 2 tablespoons ricotta, 2 zucchini slices (placed side by side or overlapping, depending on the size of the tomato slice), 2 more tablespoons ricotta, 1 more tomato slice, and 1 last rounded tablespoon of ricotta. Repeat with the remaining ingredients.

**2.** Garnish with a drizzle of balsamic vinegar and a sprinkle of basil.

### VARIATIONS

**RAW PESTO LASAGNA:** Replace the Fast Tofu Ricotta with 1 (14-ounce) block extra-firm tofu, drained, pressed, and crumbled, mixed with 1 batch Pistachio Pesto (page 226).

**RAW MEDITERRANEAN LASAGNA:** Omit the Fast Tofu Ricotta, balsamic vinegar, and basil. Use White Bean Hummus (page 43) mixed with ½ cup pitted and chopped kalamata or green olives, ½ cup chopped artichokes, and ¼ cup chopped fresh parsley. Drizzle the top with olive oil and garnish with more chopped fresh parsley.

**TIP:** *It's nice to serve salads or raw dishes like this on a chilled plate. Place your serving plates in the refrigerator at least 30 minutes before building the lasagna stacks.*

# Spaghetti Squash Primavera

GF  NF  SF

1 large spaghetti squash (roughly 4 pounds), halved and seeded

3 tablespoons olive oil, divided

1 onion, chopped

2 cups chopped broccoli florets

½ cup pitted and sliced green olives

1 cup halved cherry tomatoes

3 garlic cloves, minced

1½ teaspoons Italian seasoning

¾ teaspoon sea salt

½ teaspoon black pepper

Pine nuts, for garnish (optional)

Walnut Parmesan (page 230) or store-bought vegan Parmesan, for garnish (optional)

Red pepper flakes, for garnish (optional)

SERVES 2 TO 4 • PREP TIME: 10 MINUTES •
COOK TIME: 40 MINUTES

My dear friend Jordan used to eat spaghetti squash all the time when we lived together in a tiny apartment in Chicago. If only I had seen the light back then! I have missed years of enjoying what is truly one of the most awesome varieties of squash. Make this recipe and the variations. Once you fall in love with the simplicity of this squash, personalize it with your favorite mix-ins and sauces.

1. Preheat the oven to 400°F. Line a baking sheet with parchment paper.

2. Brush the rims and the insides of both squash halves with 1 tablespoon of olive oil. Place on the prepared baking sheet, cut-sides down. Bake for 35 to 45 minutes, until a fork can easily pierce the flesh. Set aside until cool enough to handle, 10 to 15 minutes.

3. While the squash is cooling, heat 1 tablespoon of olive oil in a large skillet over medium heat. Add the onion and broccoli and sauté for 3 minutes, or until the onion is soft. Add the olives and tomatoes and cook for an additional 3 to 5 minutes, until the broccoli is fork-tender and the tomatoes have started to wilt. Add the garlic and cook for 1 additional minute, or until fragrant. Remove from the heat.

4. Use a fork to gently pull the squash flesh from the skin and separate the flesh into strands. The strands wrap around the squash horizontally, so rake your fork in the same direction as the strands to make the longest spaghetti squash noodles.

5. Toss the noodles into the skillet with the vegetables. Add the final 1 tablespoon of olive oil, Italian seasoning, salt, and pepper and mix well to combine. Divide among bowls and garnish with pine nuts, Parmesan, and red pepper flakes, if desired.

## VARIATIONS

**SPAGHETTI SQUASH AND MEATBALLS:** Top the spaghetti squash noodles with Italian Meatballs (page 76) and Magnificent Marinara (page 231).

**SPAGHETTI SQUASH AND BROCCOLI ALFREDO:** Mix the spaghetti squash noodles with Cauliflower Alfredo Your Way (page 111) and steamed broccoli florets for a combination that is truly decadent and satisfying—and, most rewardingly, low in calories.

**TIP:** *You can also roast a spaghetti squash whole. Pierce the squash with a small, sharp knife several times, then bake as directed. It usually takes about an hour and is done when a fork can pierce through the outer peel and all the way into the interior.*

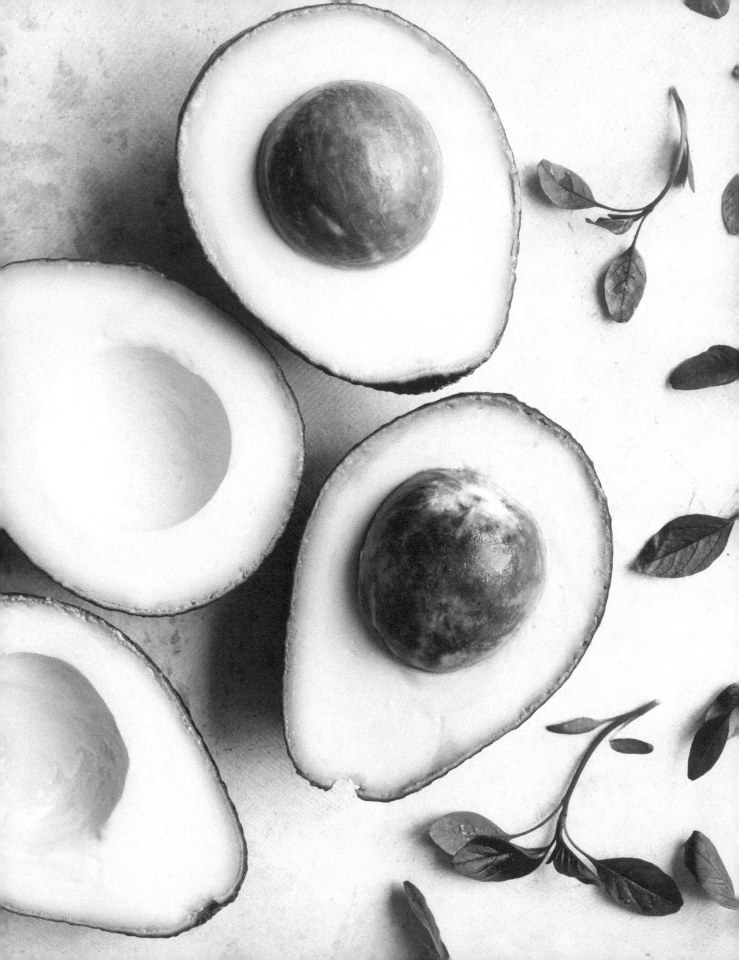

# CHAPTER 10

# Avocado

"But I'm a good fat!" screams the avocado.

I'm not going to get all science-y and in your face with health facts, but I quickly want to mention monounsaturated and polyunsaturated fats. These are unsaturated or "good fats." When consumed in moderation in place of foods that contain saturated fats, they do cool things like reduce your risk for heart disease, decrease cholesterol and blood-pressure levels, and even relieve the symptoms of arthritis. Avocados are the only fruit with monounsaturated fats, so run out and get you some.

And they're not just for toast or salads! In this chapter you will discover many ways to eat avocado, from pasta and gazpacho to breakfast pizza and even some variations on the classic guacamole. What's even better is that avocado isn't typically cooked because heat makes the texture somewhat mushy and undesirable, meaning most of these recipes are very quick.

All and all, I think it's safe to say you can't go wrong with a little avocado in your life. I hope these recipes will help you enjoy it even more.

# Avocado, Kale, and Kiwi Smoothie Bowl

**GF  NF  SF  30**

¼ avocado

1 banana, frozen

1 cup stemmed and roughly
chopped kale

2 kiwis, peeled and sliced, divided

1 cup unsweetened soy or almond milk

¼ cup fresh blackberries

1 tablespoon chia seeds

SERVES 1 • PREP TIME: 5 MINUTES

My dear friend Ashley has an amazing website, RiseShineCook.ca, that constantly inspires me to live my best life and feed myself excellent food. Her Instagram account @riseshinecook is full of vibrant, gorgeous photos and recipes that make eating whole plant-based foods look like a stroll over the rainbow. This smoothie bowl is inspired by her.

**1.** In a blender, combine the avocado, banana, kale, 1 kiwi, and milk. Blend until smooth.

**2.** Transfer the mixture to a bowl and top with the remaining kiwi and blackberries. Sprinkle with chia seeds.

### VARIATIONS

**SUPER GREEN SMOOTHIE BOWL:** Add 1 cup baby spinach and an additional ¼ cup milk to the blender.

**STRAWBERRY-BANANA BOWL:** Omit the kiwi. Add ¼ cup hulled strawberries when blending the smoothie. Add ½ banana, sliced, and another ¼ cup strawberries, hulled and sliced, on top of the bowl.

**TIP:** *For a touch of sweetness, start by adding 1 teaspoon maple syrup and add more as desired.*

# Guacamole Three Ways

 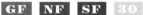  

2 avocados, peeled, pitted, and diced

1 Roma or small tomato, chopped

¼ cup minced onion

1 jalapeño pepper, minced

Juice of ½ lime

2 tablespoons chopped fresh cilantro

¼ teaspoon sea salt

¼ teaspoon black pepper

SERVES 4 TO 6 • PREP TIME: 10 MINUTES

Guacamole . . . you know it, you love it. You have consumed a party-size portion single-handedly in one sitting, and you have gazed at the last bite when out with friends and scooped it up and not apologized one bit (nor should you). And now you have this recipe with a couple of easy variations for whenever the craving strikes. So make that pitcher of margaritas and let the good times roll.

In a large bowl, mash all the ingredients with a fork or potato masher until well combined.

### VARIATIONS

**MANGO GUACAMOLE:** Replace the tomato with ¾ cup finely chopped mango.

**CHARRED CORN AND BLACK BEAN GUACAMOLE:** In a medium skillet, heat 1 tablespoon olive oil over medium heat. Sauté ½ cup corn kernels for 6 to 8 minutes, until browned. Add the corn and ½ cup canned, rinsed, and drained black beans to the avocado mixture after you have mashed it up. Mix well to combine, but take care not to mash the beans.

**TIP:** *Cilantro is a personal preference for a lot of people. When it is mixed with the right ingredients, I feel it is an essential herb. However, if you are someone who harbors a strong aversion to cilantro, you can omit it and still enjoy guacamole.*

# Avocado, Watermelon, and Feta Salad

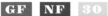  

**GF** **NF** 30

1 recipe Fast Feta (page 225)

2 cups watermelon balls or 1-inch cubes

1 avocado, peeled, pitted, and diced

1 to 2 tablespoons roughly chopped fresh mint

Mint sprigs, for garnish (optional)

SERVES 2 TO 4 • PREP TIME: 10 MINUTES

Watermelon and avocado are so refreshing! I always see them in some variation when I join friends at the park for a picnic or a backyard barbecue. Combining the two with the spices, olive oil, and lemon juice from the Fast Feta creates a salad that disappears when I bring it to social functions.

**1.** In a large bowl, combine the feta, watermelon, avocado, and 1 tablespoon of mint. Mix well to combine and add more mint if desired.

**2.** Divide among bowls and garnish each with a sprig of mint, if desired.

### VARIATIONS

**ARUGULA, WATERMELON, AND FETA SALAD:** Omit the mint and avocado. Mix the watermelon and feta with 5 ounces roughly chopped arugula until well combined.

**CUCUMBER, WATERMELON, AND FETA SALAD:** Omit the mint and avocado. Mix in 2 cups sliced mini cucumbers and 2 tablespoons chopped fresh basil.

**TIP:** *Make watermelon balls for this salad with a melon baller. I find it quicker than chopping it into cubes.*

# The Great Green Salad

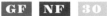  

1 head Boston or Bibb lettuce

8 asparagus spears, trimmed and cut into 2-inch pieces

2 mini seedless cucumbers, sliced

1 small zucchini, cut into ribbons with potato peeler

1 avocado, peeled, pitted, and sliced

½ cup Green Goddess Dressing (page 220) or store-bought vegan green goddess dressing

2 scallions, thinly sliced

**SERVES 4 • PREP TIME: 10 MINUTES**

You won't find a bigger fan of vegan pizza and macaroni and cheese than me. But it's all about balance. Fortunately, I have found an intense love for fresh vegetables and fruits as well. I love diving into a salad like this because I know I'm fueling my body with nutrients. And the Green Goddess Dressing is packed full of flavor that only enhances this salad's natural appeal.

Divide the lettuce leaves among 4 plates. Top each with some of the asparagus, cucumber, zucchini, and avocado. Drizzle each bowl with 2 tablespoons of dressing and sprinkle with scallions.

## VARIATIONS

**BAKED TOFU AND BACON GREEN SALAD:** Add Basic Baked Tofu (page 137) and Portobello Bacon (page 185) for a scrumptious and filling meal.

**GREEN BUDDHA BOWL:** Add Basic Baked Tofu (page 137), roasted or steamed sweet potatoes, brown rice, and alfalfa sprouts.

**TIP:** *Size doesn't matter when picking the right bunch of asparagus—thick asparagus stalks are just more mature than the thin stalks. Instead, look for bright green or violet-tinged spears with firm stems. Make sure the tips are closed and compact.*

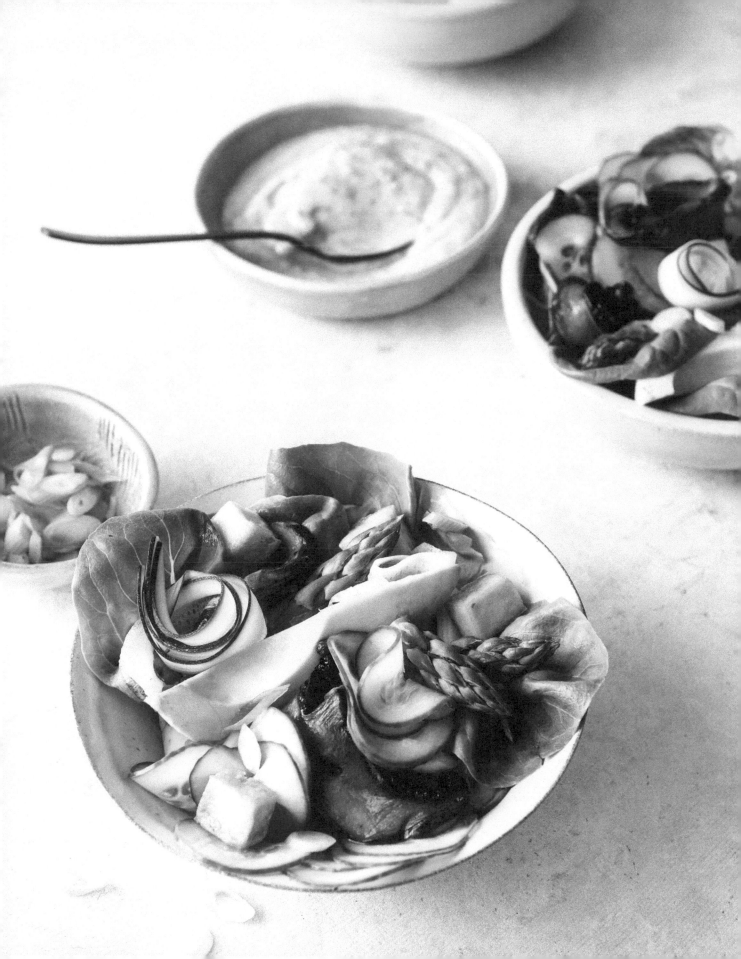

# Avocado, Cucumber, and Mint Gazpacho

**GF** **NF** **SF** **30**

1 avocado, peeled, pitted, and cubed

3 cups peeled and diced cucumber (about 2 large cucumbers)

1 cup water

2 tablespoons chopped fresh mint

Juice of 1 lemon

½ teaspoon sea salt

Fresh mint leaves, for garnish (optional)

SERVES 4 · PREP TIME: 10 MINUTES

I'm not usually a big fan of gazpacho, but this one I could eat every day. The watermelon variation is perfect for a hot summer day, and is a nice contrast to grilled foods if you are having a cookout.

**1.** In a blender, combine the avocado, cucumber, water, mint, lemon juice, and salt. Blend until smooth.

**2.** Garnish each serving with a mint leaf, if desired.

### VARIATIONS

**WATERMELON, CUCUMBER, AND MINT GAZPACHO:** Replace the avocado with 2 cups cubed watermelon.

**CUCUMBER, BASIL, AND CORN GAZPACHO:** Omit the mint. Use ¼ cup fresh basil, blend as directed, then add 1 cup corn kernels. Garnish with fresh basil leaves, if desired.

**TIP:** *Chill your cucumber, water, and lemon before blending, so the gazpacho will be cold and can be served immediately. You can refrigerate this cold soup for 1 to 4 hours before serving, but it's best eaten the day it's made.*

# Open-Faced Avocado, Bacon, and Tomato Sandwich

½ cup Lemon-Thyme Aioli (page 223) or store-bought vegan mayonnaise

4 thick slices vegan bread, toasted

1 avocado, peeled, pitted, and sliced

1 batch Portobello Bacon (page 185) or store-bought vegan bacon

1 large tomato, cut into 8 slices

Sea salt

Black pepper

SERVES 4 • PREP TIME: 10 MINUTES

Let everyone else have their BLT, we've got our ABT! A big stacked sandwich served open-faced always has my number. Even better, this one is full of delicious avocado and veggies. Serving this open-faced allows you to pile it high and not worry about these beautiful ingredients falling all over, as they would if you were eating it by hand. Grab a fork and dig in!

**1.** Spread 2 tablespoons aioli on each piece of toast.

**2.** Divide the avocado slices evenly among the toast. Top each with some bacon and 2 tomato slices. Sprinkle with salt and pepper.

### VARIATIONS

**CLASSIC BLT:** Replace the avocado with 2 lettuce leaves per sandwich (romaine, Boston, or Bibb are recommended). Toast 4 more slices of bread and make it a closed sandwich.

**SUN-DRIED TOMATO, AVOCADO, AND SPINACH PANINI:** Omit the tomato and bacon. Make 2 closed paninis. For each sandwich, start by spreading 2 tablespoons aioli on 1 slice of bread. Layer on 2 tablespoons chopped sun-dried tomatoes, some avocado slices, and ¼ cup finely chopped spinach, then top with another slice of bread. If you're using a panini press, cook for 5 to 7 minutes. If you're using a skillet, melt 1 tablespoon vegan butter over medium heat. Add the sandwich and place a heavy saucepot or skillet on top of the sandwich to weigh it down. Put something solid and heavy, like 2 cans of beans, in the pot to make it even heavier. Cook for 5 to 7 minutes per side.

**TIP:** *If you're using store-bought vegan bacon, crisp it up in a skillet according to the package directions before using it on the sandwich.*

# Stuffed Avocado

2 avocados, halved and pitted

1 (15-ounce) can black beans, rinsed and drained

1 cup frozen (and thawed) or fresh corn kernels

½ cup seeded and diced tomato

Juice of ½ lime

1 tablespoon maple syrup

1 teaspoon olive oil

2 pinches sea salt

2 pinches black pepper

1 tablespoon chopped fresh cilantro

**SERVES 4 • PREP TIME: 10 MINUTES**

There is an awesome restaurant in San Antonio called Viva Vegeria. Fred Garza, the chef and owner, serves up this massively delicious bowl of kale with a stuffed avocado. Chef Fred and his brilliance loosely inspire this super-tasty stuffed avocado, which comes together easily. My favorite variation is the one that uses Chickpea-of-the-Sea.

**1.** Scoop some avocado flesh from each half with a spoon, leaving a ¼- to ½-inch wall of avocado in the shell.

**2.** In a large bowl, mix together the scooped-out avocado, beans, corn, tomato, lime juice, maple syrup, oil, salt, pepper, and cilantro until well incorporated.

**3.** Spoon the filling into the avocado shells and enjoy.

### VARIATIONS

**CHICKPEA-OF-THE-SEA STUFFED AVOCADO:** Fill the avocado shells with the mixture from the Chickpea-of-the-Sea Sandwich (page 53). Serve atop a bed of mixed spring greens.

**LENTIL-STUFFED AVOCADO:** Fill the avocado shells with Warm Lentil Salad (page 69). Serve over sautéed chopped kale.

**TIP:** *If this is your first time pitting an avocado, check out some YouTube videos for a visual tutorial, to keep your hands safe and happy.*

# Avocado Breakfast Pizza

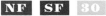 **NF** **SF** 30

2 (10-inch) flour tortillas

Nonstick cooking spray

1 avocado, peeled and pitted

Juice of ½ lime

¼ teaspoon sea salt

¼ teaspoon black pepper

¼ cup thinly sliced cherry tomatoes

¼ cup chopped fresh basil

Red pepper flakes

SERVES 2 TO 4 • PREP TIME: 5 MINUTES • COOK TIME: 10 MINUTES

Pizza: Any meal. Any time. Any place. I want it in my life every day in any form possible, and this is my favorite breakfast of all time. The crispy tortilla shell with creamy avocado mash is a dream team combination, with just a sprinkle of red pepper flakes and chopped basil to make it pop. You're welcome.

**1.** Preheat the oven to 375°F. Line a baking sheet with parchment paper.

**2.** Place the tortillas on the prepared baking sheet and lightly coat with nonstick cooking spray. Bake for 5 minutes, flip, and spray again. Bake for 3 more minutes, or until they are slightly browned and crisp.

**3.** In a medium bowl, mash the avocado with the lime juice, salt, and pepper.

**4.** Spread the avocado mash on each tortilla and top with the tomatoes. Sprinkle with basil and red pepper flakes.

### VARIATIONS

**DELUXE AVOCADO BREAKFAST PIZZA:** Top off this recipe with Scrappy Scrambler (page 138) for a heartier breakfast pizza.

**SUMMER VEGETABLE AVOCADO BREAKFAST PIZZA:** Top off this recipe with Summer Squash Skillet (page 163). You will have more than enough squash left over from the recipe; use it as a side dish for dinner.

**TIP:** *If you have ripe avocados on hand and you want to use them up, move right along to the Guacamole (page 172). Use any of those variations in place of the avocado mash in this recipe. You'll still have some left over for dip.*

# Sweet Potato Toast with Smashed Avocado

2 medium sweet potatoes, cut lengthwise into ½-inch slices

Nonstick cooking spray

Sea salt

Black pepper

2 avocados, peeled and pitted

Sriracha sauce

Chopped fresh cilantro

SERVES 2 TO 4 • PREP TIME: 10 MINUTES • COOK TIME: 10 MINUTES

Avocado toast has been all the rage for the last few years. I was doing recipe development for a restaurant whose entire goal shifted at one point to opening an avocado toast bar. Sounds amazing, right? It has yet to materialize, but you better believe I'll be the first in line if it pops up. Until then . . .

1. Preheat the oven to 450°F. Line a baking sheet with parchment paper.

2. Spread the sweet potato slices in a single layer on the prepared baking sheet. Coat both sides with nonstick cooking spray and sprinkle lightly with salt and pepper. Bake for 6 minutes, flip each slice, and bake for an additional 6 minutes.

3. While the sweet potatoes are baking, mash the avocados in a small bowl. Season with salt and pepper.

4. Divide the avocado mash among the sweet potato slices, drizzle with sriracha, sprinkle with cilantro, and serve.

### VARIATIONS

**CLASSIC AVOCADO TOAST:** Slather the avocado mash on vegan toast and top with sriracha and cilantro.

**PINEAPPLE AVOCADO TOAST:** Add 1 cup finely chopped pineapple to the avocado mash. Try peaches or mangos, too.

TIP: *Slicing a potato lengthwise can be tricky. It's important to square it off so it is flat on one side. Once it has a flat side to steady it, lay the flat side down on the cutting board and slice away with ease.*

# Veggie Avocado Carbonara

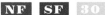  

1 pound uncooked spaghetti

1 cup frozen peas

¾ cup chopped sun-dried tomatoes

1 avocado, peeled and pitted

1¾ cups low-sodium vegetable broth

¼ cup olive oil

Juice of ½ lemon

1 teaspoon onion powder

½ teaspoon garlic powder

¾ teaspoon sea salt

¼ teaspoon black pepper

Walnut Parmesan (page 230) or
    store-bought vegan Parmesan,
    for garnish (optional)

Red pepper flakes, for garnish
    (optional)

SERVES 8 • PREP TIME: 10 MINUTES • COOK TIME: 12 MINUTES

I love miso, cashews, and nutritional yeast dearly, and you will see them frequently in chapter 13. But before then, I wanted you to have a go-to creamy pasta that doesn't require any specialty items. I think this pasta, the Sweet Potato Mac (page 132), and the Cauliflower Alfredo Your Way (page 111) totally hit the mark for that. I hope you agree.

**1.** Cook the spaghetti according to the package directions. Add the peas and sun-dried tomatoes to the boiling water with the pasta for the last 2 minutes of cooking. Drain and set aside.

**2.** While the pasta is boiling, combine the avocado, broth, oil, lemon juice, onion powder, garlic powder, salt, and pepper in a blender and blend for 1 to 2 minutes, until smooth.

**3.** Mix the cooked pasta and vegetables with the avocado-cream sauce. Divide among bowls and garnish with Parmesan and red pepper flakes, if desired.

### VARIATIONS

**MEATY AVOCADO CARBONARA:** Top with vegan chicken slices and Portobello Bacon (page 185).

**GOING GREEN AVOCADO CARBONARA:** Add 1 (10-ounce) package baby spinach when combining the pasta and sauce and stir until the spinach is wilted. The pasta must still be hot to get the spinach to wilt.

**TIP:** *When preparing spaghetti, use the biggest pot you have and submerge the pasta under the boiling water right at the start for even cooking.*

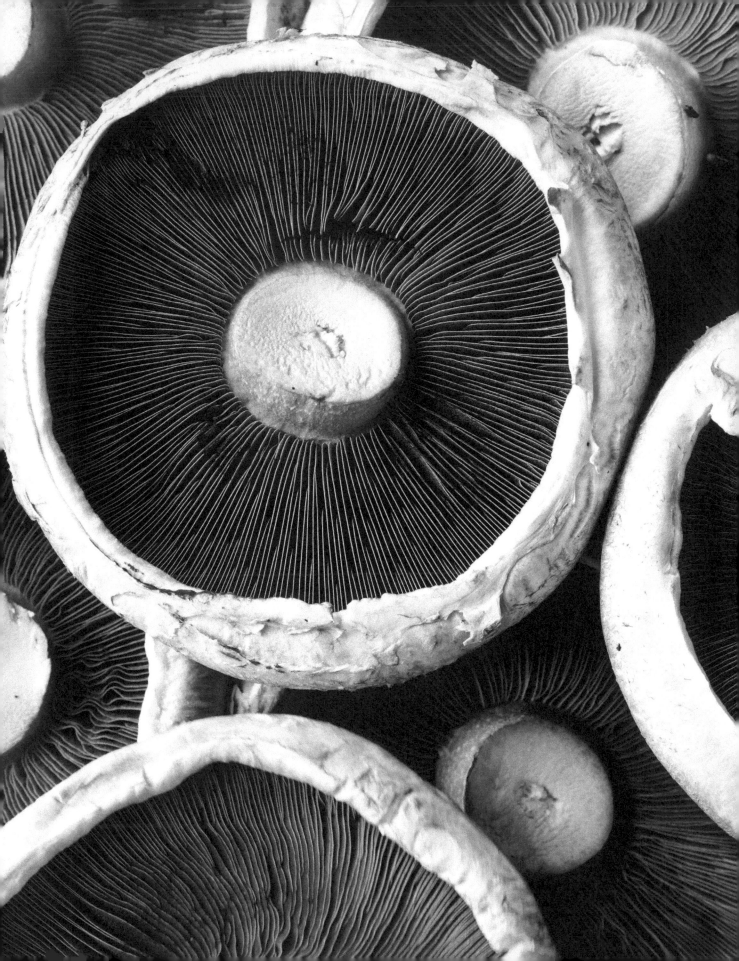

# CHAPTER 11

# Mushrooms

Mushrooms . . . the entire world has strong feelings toward these little guys. You either love them or hate them. There was a time I wasn't very fond of them, but now I can't imagine my life without them. Somewhere along the way I found a love for mushrooms and have never looked back.

There are all types of mushrooms, but we are focusing on only the three that are most commonly found at your local supermarket: portobellos, baby bellas, and white button mushrooms.

Don't get me wrong: I love shitakes, maitakes, king oysters, enokis, and so on. If you are feeling adventurous about mushrooms, I urge you to check out one of my favorite Instagram accounts, @mississippivegan. Timothy Pakron is an outstanding chef and photographer who also happens to be a master at foraging mushrooms. His account is a feast for the eyes.

But we are going basic for this chapter. If you are an avid mushroom forager, I have a suspicion you were given this book by someone who doesn't really get you.

# Portobello Bacon

**GF** **NF** 30

2 large portobello mushroom caps,
   cut into ¼-inch-thick strips

3 tablespoons olive oil

2 teaspoons soy sauce or
   gluten-free tamari

¼ teaspoon black pepper

SERVES 4 TO 6 • PREP TIME: 5 MINUTES •
COOK TIME: 25 MINUTES

Shitake bacon was my first introduction to mushroom bacon. While fresh shitakes aren't the most difficult to find, I have discovered on my travels they are not always readily available. Portobellos, on the other hand, are usually the first mushroom I see when I look at the mushroom selection at any grocery store. For that reason, I give you Portobello Bacon.

**1.** Preheat the oven to 375°F. Line a baking sheet with parchment paper.

**2.** In a medium bowl, toss the mushrooms with the oil, soy sauce, and pepper until fully coated. Spread them in a single layer on the prepared baking sheet.

**3.** Bake for 15 minutes, toss with a spatula, and bake for an additional 10 to 15 minutes, until reduced in size and darker in color. Watch closely, as the mushrooms will go from crisp to burnt very quickly.

### VARIATIONS

**SMOKED MAPLE PORTOBELLO BACON:** Omit 1 tablespoon of olive oil. Add 1 tablespoon maple syrup and ½ teaspoon liquid smoke along with the remaining 2 tablespoons of olive oil, the soy sauce, and the pepper.

**BACON AND TOMATO GRILLED CHEESE SANDWICH:** Butter 2 slices hearty vegan bread. Layer the unbuttered side of 1 slice with bacon, tomato slices, and Easy Cheese Sauce (page 224). Close with the other slice of bread, buttered-side out. Cook in a skillet over medium heat until golden brown, about 4 minutes per side.

**TIP:** *When washing mushrooms, it's important to wipe off the tops with a damp paper towel to remove any dirt and debris. Don't submerge mushrooms in water, because they will get waterlogged. The goal with this recipe is to create a crispy texture. Extra water content works against this goal.*

# Belle of the Buffalo Ball Sandwich

`30`

SERVES 4 • PREP TIME: 5 MINUTES • COOK TIME: 20 MINUTES

1 cup hot sauce (Frank's RedHot preferred)

¼ cup vegan butter, melted

4 large portobello mushroom caps, stemmed

½ teaspoon sea salt

½ teaspoon black pepper

4 romaine lettuce leaves

4 vegan hamburger buns

4 tomato slices

¼ red onion, thinly sliced

Unhidden Valley Ranch Dressing (page 221) or store-bought vegan ranch dressing

**TIP:** *Everyone loves a toasted bun. Melt 1 tablespoon vegan butter in a skillet and press the cut sides of the buns into the butter. Grill over medium-high heat until toasty; this should take 1 to 2 minutes. Melting the butter in the pan like this is an excellent way to avoid that dreaded moment of trying to spread cold butter on bread.*

I've had several versions of a Buffalo portobello sandwich at different vegan restaurants across the United States. However, I can say with confidence that my favorite is the one at Plum Bistro in Seattle. It's deep-fried, so of course it remains at the top of my list in my memory. My version is slightly healthier and allows me to bring the *Vegan Roadie* experience to your kitchen. Enjoy.

1. Preheat the oven to 425°F. Line a baking sheet with parchment paper.

2. In a small bowl, whisk together the hot sauce and butter.

3. Place the mushroom caps on the baking sheet, top-side down, and sprinkle with salt and pepper. Drizzle each cap with 2 tablespoons of the hot-sauce mixture. Bake for 10 minutes, flip, and drizzle the top sides with 1 tablespoon of the hot-sauce mixture. Bake for an additional 10 minutes, or until they have shrunk and the sauce has dried a bit on top.

4. To assemble each sandwich, place 1 lettuce leaf on the bottom bun, followed by a mushroom cap, a tomato slice, and a red-onion slice. Dress with ranch and close with the top bun.

## VARIATIONS

**BUFFALO CHICKEN RANCH SANDWICH:** Replace the mushrooms with breaded vegan chicken patties tossed in the hot-sauce mixture. Add avocado slices and ranch.

**BELLE OF THE BUFFALO BALL SALAD:** Toss together chopped romaine, shredded carrot, and store-bought vegan cheddar shreds. Slice the baked Buffalo portobellos and place atop the salad. Drizzle with ranch and garnish with chopped scallions.

# Pulled Mushroom BBQ Sandwich

 **NF** **30**

1 tablespoon olive oil

1 onion, chopped

1 (8-ounce) package baby bella or white button mushrooms, stemmed and sliced

2 garlic cloves, minced

½ cup Basic BBQ Sauce (page 232) or store-bought barbecue sauce

1 teaspoon paprika

½ teaspoon ground cinnamon

4 vegan hamburger buns

¼ red onion, thinly sliced

**SERVES 4 · PREP TIME: 10 MINUTES · COOK TIME: 20 MINUTES**

The best vegan pulled pork sandwich I have ever eaten was at a place called FüD in Kansas City, Missouri. It's made with jackfruit, and while I would love to give you a jackfruit recipe for this book, it's not that easy an ingredient to find far and wide. For that reason, I give you the mushroom version. If I'm being honest, I like this one more. I love the hearty texture.

**1.** In a large skillet, heat the oil over medium heat. Add the onion and sauté for 3 minutes, or until soft. Add the mushrooms and sauté for 5 minutes, or until reduced in size. Add the garlic and sauté for 1 additional minute, or until fragrant.

**2.** Add the barbecue sauce, paprika, and cinnamon and reduce the heat to low. Cook for 10 minutes, or until the sauce has reduced slightly.

**3.** Divide among the 4 buns and top with the sliced red onion.

### VARIATIONS

**HAWAIIAN MUSHROOM BBQ SANDWICH:** Add caramelized pineapple slices to your sandwich. To caramelize them, heat 1 teaspoon olive oil in a small skillet over medium-high heat and sauté fresh or canned pineapple rings for 4 to 6 minutes on each side, until they start to turn brown.

**FOURTH OF JULY BBQ SANDWICH:** Omit the red onion. Add Broccoli Slaw (page 109) to give this recipe a refreshing all-American crunch for your Independence Day celebration—or any day.

**TIP:** *If you're buying store-bought barbecue sauce, be diligent about reading labels. The most common non-vegan ingredient is honey, but sometimes other stuff sneaks its way in.*

# Mushroom, Quinoa, and Spinach Taquitos

**GF** **SF**

½ cup raw cashews, soaked in water overnight or boiled for 10 minutes, drained

¾ cup water

2 tablespoons Taco Seasoning (page 219) or store-bought taco seasoning

1 tablespoon olive oil

1 onion, chopped

1 (8-ounce) package baby bella mushrooms, diced small

1 cup cooked quinoa

1 (5-ounce) package baby spinach

¼ teaspoon sea salt

12 (6-inch) corn tortillas

Nonstick cooking spray

Sour Cream (page 222) or store-bought vegan sour cream, for serving

Salsa, for serving

SERVES 4 TO 6 • PREP TIME: 15 MINUTES • COOK TIME: 30 MINUTES

Taquitos don't have to be deep-fried. I'll never forget when I was doing Weight Watchers many years ago, before I went vegan, and I was yo-yo dieting to maintain my weight. I discovered a baked-burrito recipe that required using the tiniest bit of cooking oil spray to crisp up the outside, and my life was forever changed. I've carried that trick over to these tasty taquitos, and it serves its purpose well.

**1.** Preheat the oven to 425°F. Line a baking sheet with parchment paper.

**2.** Combine the cashews, water, and taco seasoning in a blender and blend until smooth, about 2 minutes.

**3.** Heat the oil in a large skillet over medium-high heat. Add the onion and mushrooms and sauté for 5 minutes, or until the mushrooms reduce in size. Add the quinoa, spinach, and salt and sauté for an additional 3 minutes, or until the spinach is wilted. Reduce the heat to medium-low. Pour the cashew mixture into the skillet, stir until well combined, and remove from the heat.

**4.** Lay the corn tortillas in a double layer on the prepared baking sheet. Bake for 2 minutes. Transfer to a large plate. Leave the oven on.

**5.** To assemble the taquitos, place 1 tortilla on a flat surface. Put 2 heaping tablespoons of mushroom filling on the side of the tortilla closest to you and roll upward, away from you. Place the taquito, seam-side down, on the baking sheet. Repeat with the remaining tortillas and filling. Spray the taquitos with nonstick cooking spray and bake for 18 minutes, or until golden brown.

**6.** Serve warm with sour cream and salsa on the side.

**KALE AND SWEET POTATO TAQUITOS:** Use Kale and Sweet Potato Hash (page 33) as a taquito filling. Mix with the cashew mixture and continue with the recipe as written.

**SOYRIZO TAQUITOS:** Replace the quinoa with store-bought soy chorizo. Game changer.

TIP: *Trader Joe's has the most amazing soy chorizo I have ever had. If you are fortunate enough to have a Trader Joe's in your neck of the woods, do yourself a favor and throw a package into your shopping cart for this recipe the next time you make it.*

# Quick Thai Coconut Mushroom Soup

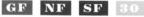

1½ cups low-sodium vegetable broth, divided

2 garlic cloves, minced

1 tablespoon minced fresh ginger

1 (8-ounce) package baby bella or white button mushrooms, stemmed and sliced

1 (13.5-ounce) can full-fat coconut milk

Juice of ½ lemon

Juice of ½ lime

2 tablespoons chopped fresh Thai basil

1 tablespoon chopped fresh cilantro

Fresh cilantro leaves, for garnish (optional)

Lime wedges, for garnish (optional)

SERVES 4 · PREP TIME: 5 MINUTES · COOK TIME: 10 MINUTES

This soup is inspired by *tom kha gai* (Thai coconut chicken soup). Most recipes have a lengthy list of ingredients, including the specialty items of lemongrass and lime leaf. I created this super-simple soup that can easily be tossed together with stuff you have on hand or after a breezy trip to the grocery store on your way home from work. To make it even easier, if you can't find Thai basil, use regular basil this time around.

1. Heat ½ cup of broth in a large saucepot over medium-high heat. Sauté the garlic and ginger in the broth for 1 minute, or until fragrant.

2. Add the mushrooms and slowly pour in the remaining 1 cup of broth. Bring to a boil and reduce the heat to a simmer.

3. Add the coconut milk, lemon juice, lime juice, basil, and chopped cilantro. Let simmer for 5 minutes, or until heated through.

4. Garnish with whole cilantro leaves and lime wedges, if desired.

## VARIATIONS

**SPICY RED CURRY COCONUT SOUP:** Add 1 to 3 teaspoons Thai red curry paste when adding the coconut milk. Adjust to your desired heat level.

**COCONUT CHICKEN AND MUSHROOM SOUP:** Add 1 cup chopped or shredded vegan chicken. At the start of the recipe, before you do anything else, heat 1 teaspoon toasted sesame oil or olive oil in a skillet over medium-high heat, add the chicken, and sauté for 3 minutes, or until slightly browned. Continue with the recipe as written.

**TIP:** *This soup is very gentle with flavors. It doesn't require much actual cooking, so be careful not to pull a "set it and forget it" move and walk away for 30 minutes while it's simmering. Your liquid will cook away in that time and you won't be left with much soup.*

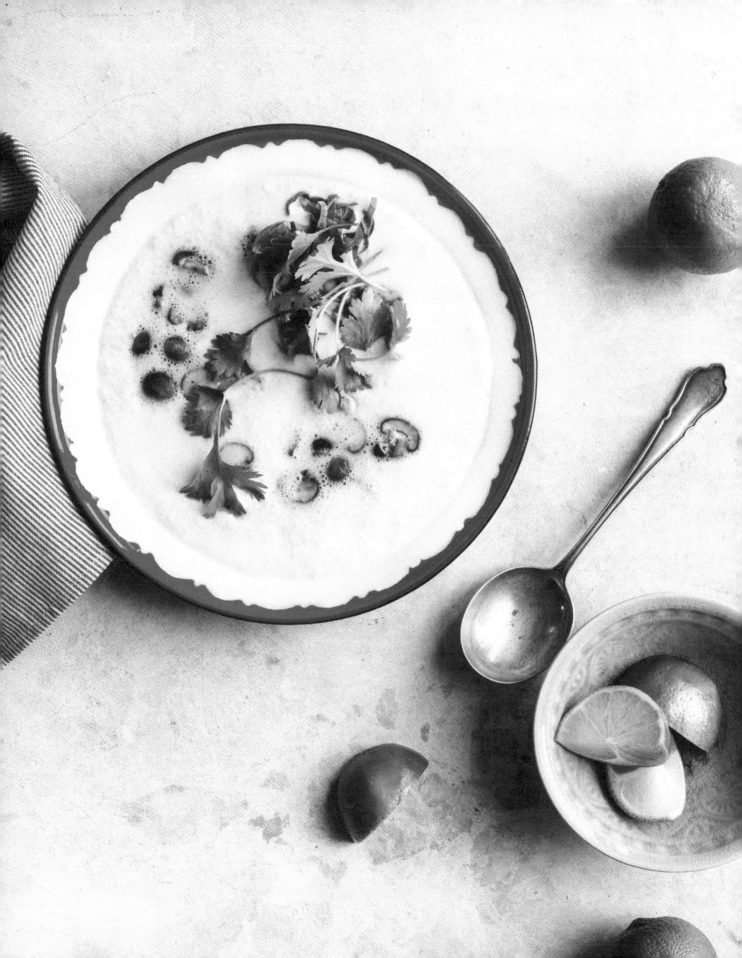

# Drunken Mushroom Noodles

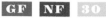

8 ounces uncooked wide rice noodles

3 tablespoons toasted sesame oil, divided

½ cup sliced onion

1 green bell pepper, seeded and sliced

4 (8-ounce) packages baby bella or white button mushrooms, stemmed and sliced

2 tablespoons chili garlic sauce

2 tablespoons soy sauce or gluten-free tamari

Juice of ½ lime

1 cup chopped fresh Thai basil, divided

SERVES 6 · PREP TIME: 10 MINUTES · COOK TIME: 15 MINUTES

Thai food is delicious and can be ordered vegan-style with confidence in most restaurants. The key is asking them to leave out the fish sauce, oyster sauce, and eggs. There are also completely vegan Thai restaurants, like Araya's Place in Seattle, one of my favorites. I get the drunken noodles every time. This is a super-simple spin on one of my favorite Thai dishes.

**1.** Prepare the pasta according to the package directions. Drain and toss with 1 tablespoon of sesame oil and set aside.

**2.** In a large skillet, heat 1 tablespoon of sesame oil over medium heat. Add the onion and bell pepper and sauté for 5 minutes, or until soft. Add the remaining 1 tablespoon of sesame oil and the mushrooms. Cook for 5 minutes, or until the mushrooms have reduced in size.

**3.** Add the chili garlic sauce, soy sauce, and lime juice. Cook for 2 minutes, until heated through. Add the rice noodles and ½ cup of basil. Toss well to combine.

**4.** Divide among plates and garnish with the remaining ½ cup basil.

### VARIATIONS

**DRUNKEN GREENS:** Omit the rice noodles. Wilt down 2 bunches collard greens, stemmed and chopped, when heating the sauce. Cook the greens for 4 minutes, or until completely wilted.

**BEEFY DRUNKEN LO MEIN:** Replace the rice noodles with lo mein noodles. Add 2 cups vegan beef tips or chopped seitan and 1 additional tablespoon of oil with the mushrooms.

**TIP:** *If you can't find chili garlic sauce, mix 1 tablespoon sriracha sauce with 2 garlic cloves, minced. You can also substitute regular basil for the Thai basil.*

# Mindful Mushroom Stroganoff

1 tablespoon olive oil

1 onion, chopped

2 (8-ounce) packages baby bella or white button mushrooms, stemmed and sliced

4 garlic cloves, minced

¼ cup low-sodium vegetable broth

1 teaspoon paprika

½ teaspoon sea salt

½ teaspoon black pepper

¼ cup Sour Cream (page 222) or store-bought vegan sour cream

4 tablespoons chopped fresh parsley, divided

1 pound pasta of your choice, cooked

SERVES 6 • PREP TIME: 10 MINUTES • COOK TIMES: 15 MINUTES

Hamburger Helper made its way to the dinner table frequently when I was growing up. My favorite kind was always the stroganoff. You'll see here that it's easy to create that decadent sauce without cream.

**1.** Heat the oil in a large skillet over medium heat. Add the onion and mushrooms and sauté for 5 to 8 minutes, until the mushrooms are soft and have reduced in size. Add the garlic and sauté for 1 additional minute, or until fragrant. Add the broth, paprika, salt, and pepper and cook for 5 more minutes, or until well incorporated and heated through.

**2.** Remove from the heat and stir in the sour cream and 2 tablespoons of parsley.

**3.** Toss with the cooked pasta, divide into 6 portions, and sprinkle with the remaining 2 tablespoons of parsley.

### VARIATIONS

**STROGANOFF HELPER:** Take it back to the old days and create your very own Hamburger Helper Stroganoff. Add 1 (12-ounce) package vegan beef crumbles to the skillet, along with an extra tablespoon of olive oil, when adding the vegetable broth and spices.

**VEGETABLE TOFU STROGANOFF:** Omit the pasta and add your favorite vegetables instead. Keep things simple with 1 (10-ounce) bag frozen vegetable medley, prepared according to the package directions. If you are feeling fresh, get your favorite fresh vegetables and steam or sauté them. Serve over Basic Baked Tofu (page 137).

**TIP:** *Cashew-based sauce recipes thicken when they sit. If you make this dish ahead and use the cashew version of sour cream in this book, add a couple of tablespoons of water to loosen the sauce to the desired consistency when you reheat it.*

# Creamy Spinach-Stuffed Mushrooms

**GF** **NF**

1 tablespoon olive oil

1 onion, chopped

3 garlic cloves, minced

1 (14-ounce) block extra-firm tofu, drained and crumbled

1 (5-ounce) package baby spinach

2 teaspoons Italian seasoning

1 teaspoon onion powder

½ teaspoon garlic powder

1 teaspoon sea salt

½ teaspoon black pepper

4 large portobello mushroom caps, stemmed

**SERVES 4 • PREP TIME: 10 MINUTES • COOK TIME: 25 MINUTES**

It took me a long time to channel my inner love for mushrooms. For that reason, I'm very understanding when someone declares their dislike. But recipes like this, with a delicious, creamy filling baked until it's piping hot and slightly browned on top, have won converts time and time again. Maybe this recipe will speak to the mushroom hater in your life.

**1.** Preheat the oven to 450°F. Line a baking sheet with parchment paper.

**2.** In a large skillet, heat the oil over medium heat. Add the onion and sauté for 3 minutes, or until soft. Add the garlic and sauté for 1 additional minute, or until fragrant.

**3.** Stir in the crumbled tofu and spinach and cook for 3 minutes, or until the spinach is wilted. Add the Italian seasoning, onion powder, garlic powder, salt, and pepper and mix until well combined.

**4.** Set the mushroom caps on the prepared baking sheet, top-sides down. Divide the tofu mixture among the 4 mushroom caps. Bake for 15 to 20 minutes, until the stuffing has browned slightly.

## VARIATIONS

**SPINACH-ARTICHOKE STUFFED MUSHROOMS:** Replace the tofu mixture with the mixture from the Simple Spinach and Artichoke Flatbread (page 23) recipe.

**ROASTED-BEET STUFFED MUSHROOMS:** Replace the tofu mixture with the beet mixture from the Fancy-Free Beet Tartare with Creamy Pine Nut Ricotta (page 124) recipe. After they bake, top the mushrooms with the creamy pine nut ricotta from the same recipe.

**TIP:** *These are awesome for a party appetizer. Get baby bellas instead of large portobellos, remove the stems, and create miniature stuffed mushrooms for your guests.*

# Portobello Fajitas

 **NF** **30**

2 tablespoons soy sauce or gluten-free tamari

1 tablespoon olive oil

Juice of 2 limes

2 tablespoons chopped fresh cilantro

1 teaspoon ground cumin

1 teaspoon garlic powder

2 large portobello mushroom caps, stemmed and sliced

1 yellow bell pepper, seeded and sliced

1 red bell pepper, seeded and sliced

1 onion, halved and sliced

12 (6-inch) flour tortillas, warmed (see Tip)

Romaine lettuce, shredded, for serving (optional)

Guacamole (page 172), for serving (optional)

Sour Cream (page 222) or store-bought vegan sour cream, for serving (optional)

Easy Cheese Sauce (page 224) or store-bought vegan cheese shreds, for serving (optional)

SERVES 6 • PREP TIME: 10 MINUTES • COOK TIME: 8 MINUTES

Fajitas are always a satisfying go-to in my home. They are warm and delicious, and they fill you up. I like to put all the toppings on mine, piling it high with guacamole, sour cream, lettuce, and shredded vegan cheese. But the best thing about a fajita is you can do it your way.

**1.** In a medium bowl, mix together the soy sauce, oil, lime juice, cilantro, cumin, and garlic powder. Add the mushrooms and marinate for 10 minutes.

**2.** Add the bell peppers and onion to the mushroom bowl and combine until all the vegetables are coated.

**3.** Heat a large skillet over medium heat. Add the contents of the bowl, including the marinade, and cook for 8 minutes, or until the vegetables are tender and the liquid has been absorbed.

**4.** Serve with warm tortillas and all the toppings.

## VARIATIONS

**GARDEN GRAZER FAJITAS:** Add 1 cup chopped broccoli florets and ½ cup shredded carrot to the marinating bowl.

**PORTOBELLO BURRITOS:** Use 6 (10-inch) burrito-size tortillas instead of the corn tortillas. Add the lettuce, guacamole, and vegan cheese shreds to the fajita mixture, plus some refried vegan beans, and mix well. Divide evenly among the tortillas. Roll up each tortilla nice and tight and top with vegan sour cream and salsa.

**TIP:** *Here's an easy and quick way to gently warm tortillas: Preheat the oven to 375°F. Lay the tortillas on a baking sheet, bake for 2 minutes, transfer to a plate, and cover with an inverted plate to keep them warm.*

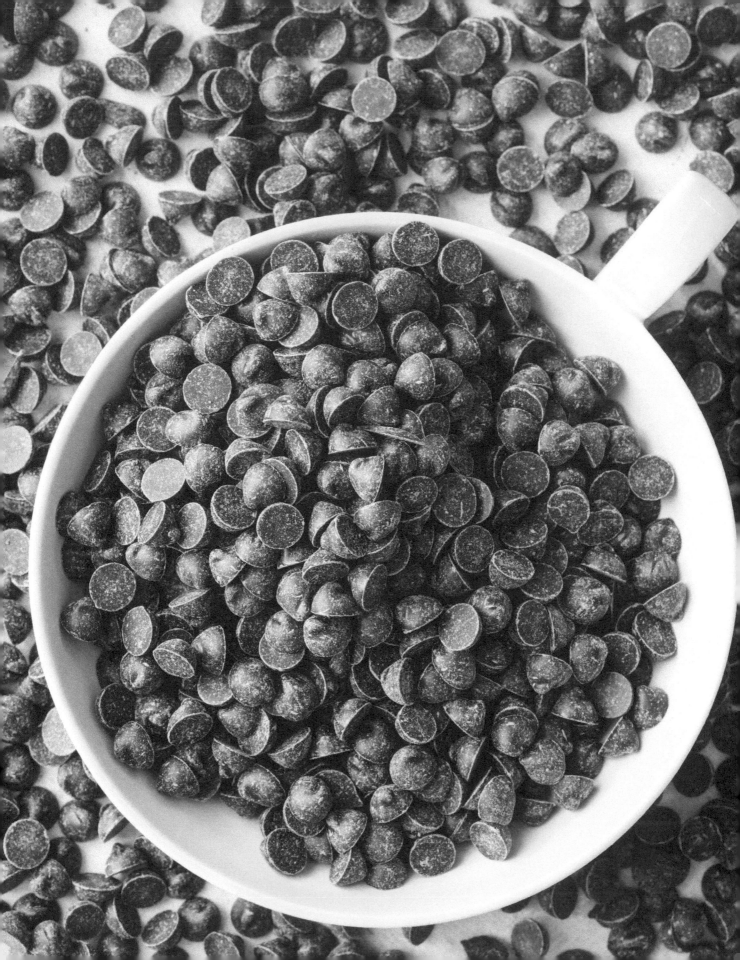

# CHAPTER 12

# Simple Sweets

Okay, you caught me—I'm aware that sweets are not an essential ingredient. But I simply could not write a cookbook without a chapter dedicated to something everyone needs to do from time to time: Treat yo' self! My sweet tooth has its own zip code, it takes up that much of my appetite. Sometimes I wish my sweet tooth would listen to my wisdom tooth when it tells me not to grab that second cupcake. But because of my sweet tooth (or shall we say teeth?), I was able to compile some of my favorite, and also very simple, sweet treats for you.

The methods for the recipes in this chapter are quick, straightforward, and easy to follow. However, some of them require baking and cooling, while others require overnight refrigeration to set. Be sure to read the directions all the way through before you start cooking a recipe, so you set aside enough time. And don't worry; some are ready to enjoy right away.

This is not strictly a dessert chapter because, let's face it, sweets are not just for after dinner. Some of these are perfect for brunch, or a midday treat. I personally love a cupcake for breakfast on the morning of my birthday. You can totally judge me, but it's my birthday and I'll do what I want.

# Watermelon-Banana Granita

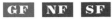

**3 bananas**
**3 cups cubed watermelon**
**Juice of 2 limes**

SERVES 8 · PREP TIME: 5 MINUTES, PLUS OVERNIGHT TO FREEZE

Popsicles are an obsession of mine. On a hot summer day there is nothing better than some flavored ice. You can certainly pop this recipe into popsicle molds if you have them, or you can enjoy it spooned out into a bowl. No ice cream machine needed—all that is required is a blender. The texture is a bit icier, but it does the trick when you need a cold sweet.

**1.** In a blender, combine all the ingredients and blend until smooth. Transfer to a 1-quart container, cover, and freeze overnight.

**2.** When ready to serve, thaw for 10 minutes and then use a sturdy spoon to scrape the desired portion from the container. Transfer to a bowl to create a shaved-ice effect.

### VARIATIONS

**BERRY-BANANA GRANITA:** Omit the watermelon. Blend the bananas and lime juice with 1 cup fresh raspberries, 1 cup fresh strawberries, 1 cup fresh blackberries, and ¼ cup orange juice.

**TROPICAL GRANITA:** Omit the watermelon and lime juice. Blend the bananas with 1 cup fresh mango chunks, 1 cup fresh pineapple chunks, 1 cup fresh peach chunks, ¼ cup orange juice, and the juice of 2 lemons.

**TIP:** *The fruit used in the variations is not as juicy as watermelon, so you will have to stop the blender and scrape down the sides to shift the contents around in your blender and get it moving a little. If you find it's not moving, add more orange juice by the tablespoon until it does.*

# Coconut–Banana Pudding

**GF** **NF** **SF**

3 bananas, divided

1 (13.5-ounce) can full-fat coconut milk

¼ cup organic cane sugar

1 tablespoon cornstarch

1 teaspoon vanilla extract

2 pinches sea salt

6 drops natural yellow food coloring (optional)

Ground cinnamon, for garnish

SERVES 4 • PREP TIME: 4 MINUTES, PLUS OVERNIGHT TO SET • COOK TIME: 5 MINUTES

Pudding makes us think of good times as a kid—a Snack Pack perhaps? For me, I think about a delicious treat at a very popular non-vegan New York City bakery. I used to get the classic banana pudding there all the time. Then I went vegan, and I quickly came up with this super-simple version that I'm delighted to share with you now.

**1.** Combine 1 banana, the coconut milk, sugar, cornstarch, vanilla, and salt in a blender. Blend until smooth and creamy. If you're using the food coloring, add it to the blender now and blend until the color is evenly dispersed.

**2.** Transfer to a saucepot and bring to a boil over medium-high heat. Immediately reduce to a simmer and whisk for 3 minutes, or until the mixture thickens to a thin pudding and sticks to a spoon.

**3.** Transfer the mixture to a container and allow to cool for 1 hour. Cover and refrigerate overnight to set.

**4.** When you're ready to serve, slice the remaining 2 bananas and build individual servings as follows: pudding, banana slices, pudding, and so on until a single-serving dish is filled to the desired level. Sprinkle with ground cinnamon.

### VARIATIONS

**CHOCOLATE MOUSSE:** Omit the bananas and cinnamon. Combine the coconut milk, cane sugar, cornstarch, and sea salt with ¼ cup fair-trade unsweetened cocoa powder and ½ teaspoon vanilla extract. Blend until smooth, then transfer to a saucepot and follow the recipe as directed.

**PUDDING OR MOUSSE PARFAIT:** Create a parfait with layers of pudding or mousse. Use fresh berries and Cinnamon Toast Crunch Granola (page 87) to create layers, and top with Coconut Whipped Cream (page 202).

**TIP:** *Bananas oxidize once peeled, making this mixture turn gray as it sits, so you'll want to eat it within 3 days. I suggest the optional food coloring if you're serving this to guests.*

# Affogato Float

30

2 scoops vegan vanilla or coffee ice cream

3 tablespoons freshly brewed or instant espresso

3 tablespoons unsweetened soy or almond milk

Sparkling water

**SERVES 1 • PREP TIME: 5 MINUTES**

I fell in love with affogato when I was filming an episode of *The Vegan Roadie* at Dulce Vegan Bakery and Cafe in Atlanta, Georgia. Affogato is a coffee-based dessert, typically a scoop of vanilla ice cream or gelato drowned in a shot of espresso. But The Cookie Counter in Seattle took it a step further: an affogato float. Yes. YAS. YESSSS. I was instantly inspired to create a recipe that allows me to indulge in this delight in my own home.

In a tall glass, combine the ice cream, espresso, and milk. Top off with sparkling water. Enjoy with a spoon.

### VARIATIONS

**VEGAN ROOT BEER FLOAT:** Use vanilla ice cream. Omit the espresso, milk, and sparkling water. Fill the glass with your favorite root beer.

**ORANGE CREAMSICLE FLOAT:** Use vanilla ice cream. Omit the espresso, milk, and sparkling water. Fill the glass with your favorite orange soda. I prefer Virgil's orange cream soda for this recipe.

**TIP:** *For a more robust flavor, go with the coffee ice cream.*

# Rainbow Sprinkle Pancakes with Coconut Whipped Cream

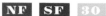 

**SERVES 4 · PREP TIME: 10 MINUTES · COOK TIME: 15 MINUTES**

**FOR THE WHIPPED CREAM**

1 (13.5-ounce) can full-fat coconut milk, refrigerated overnight

½ cup organic confectioners' sugar

**FOR THE PANCAKES**

1 cup all-purpose flour

1 tablespoon baking powder

1 tablespoon organic cane sugar

½ teaspoon sea salt

¼ teaspoon ground cinnamon

1 cup unsweetened soy or almond milk

4 tablespoons vegan rainbow cake sprinkles, divided

Canola oil, for greasing

I used to inhale Funfetti cupcakes as a kid. You know the kind made out of a box? I haven't touched those in years, but these pancakes remind me why I loved them so much: They have rainbow sprinkles, they are festive, and they are downright delicious.

*To make the whipped cream:* Open the chilled can of coconut milk and spoon out the solid portion into a small bowl. Mash the solids down with a fork, then whisk in the confectioners' sugar until smooth. Return to the refrigerator.

**1.** *To make the pancakes:* In a large bowl, whisk together the flour, baking powder, sugar, salt, and cinnamon.

**2.** Add the milk to the flour mixture and mix until just combined; do not overmix. Fold 3 tablespoons of the vegan rainbow cake sprinkles into the batter.

**3.** Lightly grease a large nonstick griddle or skillet with canola oil and warm over medium heat. For each pancake, pour ¼ cup of batter onto the warmed skillet. When bubbles start to appear in the middle, after about 2 minutes, flip the pancake and let it cook on the other side until lightly browned and cooked through, about 2 more minutes. Repeat with the remaining batter, adding more oil to the skillet as needed.

**4.** Divide the pancakes among 4 plates and top with a dollop of chilled coconut whipped cream. Finish them off with some of the remaining sprinkles.

## VARIATIONS

**WHITE-CHOCOLATE RASPBERRY PANCAKES:** Special ingredient alert: These pancakes require vegan white-chocolate chips. Plan ahead and order them online (see Tip), as you won't likely find them in your local supermarket. But these are so good that I had to include them. Add ⅓ cup vegan white-chocolate chips or chopped-up vegan white chocolate to the batter. Make a super-simple raspberry syrup by blending ½ cup maple syrup with ½ cup fresh raspberries in a blender until smooth. Drizzle this goodness on that goodness and devour.

**BANANA-STRAWBERRY PANCAKES:** Mash 1 ½ sliced bananas into the batter. Make a strawberry syrup by blending ½ cup maple syrup with ½ cup hulled and sliced fresh strawberries in a blender until smooth. Top the pancakes with the remaining ½ banana, thinly sliced, along with ¼ cup hulled and sliced strawberries. Drizzle with the strawberry syrup.

**TIP:** *My favorite brand of vegan white chocolate chips is King David White Choco Chips. I order them on Amazon. Some other recommended brands of white chocolate bars and chips are iChoc White Vanilla bar, Organica White Bar, and Pascha Organic Rice Milk White Chocolate Chips.*

*The fruit syrup in both variations will be seedy. For a smoother syrup, press the blended syrup through a fine-mesh strainer.*

# Kettle Corn

GF  NF  SF  30

½ cup popcorn kernels

¼ cup canola oil

⅓ cup organic cane sugar

1 teaspoon sea salt

**TIP:** *Do not let the kettle corn sit over the heat longer than directed, as it will stick to the pan and burn when the sugar begins to caramelize. That's the same reason you need to keep it movin' and shakin' once it starts to pop.*

SERVES 6 • PREP TIME: 5 MINUTES • COOK TIME: 5 MINUTES

Everyone I have ever dated has uttered the words "Will you make your popcorn?" when we have settled in for a movie night. The trick of it is . . . there is no trick. It's freaking easy! Though you do have to pay attention to when to pull it off the heat, or else you will have some burnt kernels. The smell of burning popcorn and the sound of fire trucks never got anyone to third base.

**1.** Combine all the ingredients in a medium saucepot. Cover and heat over medium-high heat. When the kernels start to pop, shake the pot back and forth until the popcorn has begun to rapidly pop.

**2.** After 30 seconds of continuous popping, remove the pot from the heat and continue to shake as it finishes popping. Popping will slow to 1 to 3 seconds between pops when it's ready. This all happens quickly once the kernels start to pop. The process, start to finish, takes 3 to 5 minutes.

**3.** Immediately transfer the popcorn to a bowl. Let it cool for 10 minutes, then break it apart gently with a spatula.

## VARIATIONS

**MOVIE-THEATER POPCORN:** Omit the sugar. Pop the popcorn over medium-high heat until it has filled the pot three-quarters of the way up. Turn off the heat and let it sit, covered, for an additional minute as it finishes popping. Adjust the salt to your taste. I suggest starting with only ½ teaspoon sea salt before popping, and adding more after it's popped, if desired.

**S'MORES POPCORN:** Use only 2 tablespoons canola oil and omit the sugar. After popping, toss the popcorn in a bowl with 2 tablespoons melted vegan butter, 5 crumbled graham crackers, and 1 cup vegan mini marshmallows. (Dandies is my tried and true brand of choice for vegan marshmallows.) Spread the mixture evenly on a baking sheet and allow to cool. Drizzle with ½ cup melted vegan chocolate chips and leave for 10 minutes for the chocolate to set, or else you will have a mess when you go for a handful. Transfer to a bowl and enjoy.

# Olive Oil Brownies

**NF** **SF**

Nonstick cooking spray

¾ cup all-purpose flour

¾ cup organic cane sugar

½ cup fair-trade unsweetened cocoa powder

1 tablespoon cornstarch

1 teaspoon baking powder

½ teaspoon sea salt

½ cup unsweetened soy or almond milk

½ cup olive oil

1 teaspoon vanilla extract

**TIP:** *If you are impatient like me and you struggle waiting for the brownies to cool, you can attempt to gently pop them out with a flexible spatula . . . or you can just take a fork and go to town. Who needs a portioned amount of a brownie, anyway?*

MAKES 9 • PREP TIME: 5 MINUTES • COOK TIME: 30 MINUTES

Brownies give me life. They are so simple to toss together for a delightful indulgence, and I almost always have all the ingredients on hand. In-laws dropping by and you have nothing to feed them? Olive oil brownies. Heading to a potluck that you spaced about? Olive oil brownies. Responsible for your kid's contribution to a school function? Olive oil brownies. Got lazy about cleaning the house while your partner was away on a business trip? Olive oil brownies. They fix everything.

**1.** Preheat the oven to 375°F. Lightly coat an 8-inch-square baking pan with nonstick cooking spray.

**2.** In a large bowl, whisk together the flour, sugar, cocoa powder, cornstarch, baking powder, and salt.

**3.** In a medium bowl, mix together the almond milk, oil, and vanilla. Add the liquid mixture to the dry mixture and mix until well combined. Be mindful not to overmix; this batter will be thick.

**4.** Transfer to the prepared baking pan and bake for 30 minutes, or until the top is dry and a toothpick inserted in the center comes out clean. (These brownies will be lighter in color than the usual brownie.) Cool completely before cutting.

### VARIATIONS

**FUDGY OLIVE OIL BROWNIES:** Add 1 cup vegan chocolate chips to the batter after the dry and wet ingredients have been mixed together.

**CREAM CHEESE OLIVE OIL BROWNIES:** After transferring the batter to the baking pan, dollop 6 tablespoons vegan cream cheese in various places in the batter. Run a butter knife through the cream-cheese dollops to spread them out through the batter, but not completely mix in. Bake as directed. The cream cheese will brown slightly on the edges.

# Soft-Batch Chocolate Chip Cookies

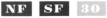 **NF** **SF** 30

2½ cups all-purpose flour

1 cup dark-brown sugar

½ cup organic cane sugar

2 tablespoons cornstarch

1 teaspoon baking soda

1 teaspoon sea salt, plus more for sprinkling

1 cup canola oil

½ cup unsweetened applesauce

2 teaspoons vanilla extract

1½ cups vegan chocolate chips

**MAKES 32 • PREP TIME: 10 MINUTES • COOK TIME: 20 MINUTES**

I should never under any circumstances be left alone with unbaked chocolate-chip-cookie dough. I just can't resist it. And I know I'm not the only one with this problem. I do hope some of this recipe makes it into your oven, so you can enjoy the soft, chewy goodness of these cookies. The result is worth resisting the raw-cookie-dough temptation.

**1.** Preheat the oven to 350°F. Line 2 baking sheets with parchment paper.

**2.** In a large bowl, whisk together the flour, sugar, cane sugar, cornstarch, baking soda, and salt until well combined. Add the canola oil, applesauce, and vanilla. Mix until a thick dough forms. Fold in the chocolate chips until they're evenly dispersed.

**3.** Form balls with 1 heaping tablespoon of dough. Place on the prepared baking sheet at least 2 inches apart and sprinkle the tops with salt.

**4.** Bake for 10 to 12 minutes, until the cookies have spread slightly and the centers appear to be set, with the edges just starting to brown. Repeat until all the dough is baked.

**5.** Let cool on a wire rack for at least 10 minutes before enjoying.

### VARIATIONS

**TRAIL-MIX COOKIES:** Use only ½ cup chocolate chips. Add ½ cup dried cranberries and ½ cup chopped pecans or walnuts when adding the chocolate chips.

**PEANUT BUTTER CHOCOLATE CHIP COOKIES:** Use only 1½ cups flour. Add 1 cup creamy peanut butter when adding the wet ingredients.

**TIP:** *I know it's hard, but try to let these cookies cool for at least 10 minutes before digging in. They set nicely in that time. But hey, I confess I'm not the person to give advice here—I'm lucky if the dough gets to the baking sheet.*

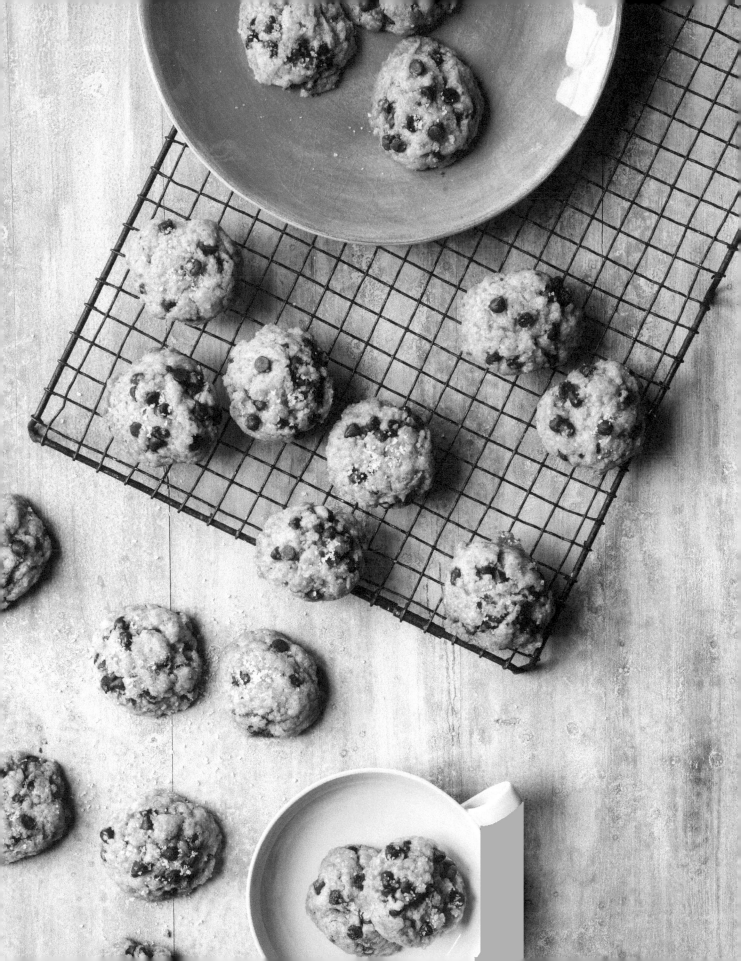

# Churro French Toast

**NF** 30

½ cup unsweetened soy or almond milk

¼ cup silken or soft tofu

1½ teaspoons vanilla extract

Pinch sea salt

½ cup organic cane sugar

1 tablespoon ground cinnamon

4 tablespoons vegan butter, divided

8 pieces sturdy vegan bread (not standard white bread)

Maple syrup, for serving

**SERVES 4 • PREP TIME: 10 MINUTES • COOK TIME: 15 MINUTES**

*Churro:* a sweet snack consisting of a strip of fried dough dusted with sugar or cinnamon. *French toast:* bread that is coated and fried. Basically, I combined the two. You're welcome.

**1.** In a wide, shallow bowl, whisk together the milk, tofu, vanilla, and salt, making sure to break down the tofu, until the mixture is smooth.

**2.** In another wide, shallow bowl, whisk together the sugar and cinnamon until well combined.

**3.** Heat a large skillet over medium-high heat. Drop 1 tablespoon of butter into the pan. As it melts, quickly dredge 2 pieces of bread through the milk mixture, being sure to get only the outsides of the bread moist. Do not soak it.

**4.** Transfer both slices of bread to the skillet and cook until lightly browned, about 2 minutes per side. Transfer the bread to the sugar-and-cinnamon mixture and coat evenly on both sides, knocking off any excess sugar and cinnamon.

**5.** Repeat with the remaining bread, 2 pieces at a time, melting 1 tablespoon of butter to start each time. Serve hot, topped with maple syrup.

**VARIATIONS**

**BANANA-STUFFED FRENCH TOAST:** Omit the sugar-and-cinnamon mixture. Build the stuffed French toast with 1 piece of French toast on a plate, followed by ¼ to ½ cup Coconut-Banana Pudding (page 200) and a layer of freshly sliced bananas, topped with another piece of French toast and a sprinkle of cinnamon.

**CLASSIC FRENCH TOAST:** Omit the sugar-and-cinnamon mixture. Add ½ teaspoon ground cinnamon and ¼ teaspoon ground nutmeg to the milk mixture. Serve with vegan butter and maple syrup on the side.

**TIP:** *Tongs are incredibly useful for this recipe when coating the pieces of French toast with the sugar-and-cinnamon mixture. In terms of "sturdy bread," I'm referring to crusty loaves, direct from a baker if possible. For the best results, you want "country" or "farm" bread that is thick and chewy, the opposite of standard white bread. Packaged is fine, too; again, look for thick slices to avoid the typical sogginess that can make for disappointing French toast.*

# Luscious Lemon Squares
# with Coconut Shortbread Crust

NF SF

Nonstick cooking spray

1 cup all-purpose flour

⅓ cup coconut oil

½ cup organic confectioners' sugar, plus more for dusting

½ cup freshly squeezed lemon juice (about 4 lemons)

½ cup unsweetened soy or almond milk

1 cup organic cane sugar

1 teaspoon vanilla extract

½ cup water

3 tablespoons cornstarch

MAKES 16 • PREP TIME: 10 MINUTES, PLUS OVERNIGHT TO SET • COOK TIME: 10 MINUTES

When I make these lemon squares for a gathering, I have to wrap the pan tightly in plastic wrap so I don't eat them all before they leave the apartment. They're so decadent yet light, it's easy to overindulge, so best to make them when you know you will have company to share them with.

**1.** Preheat the oven to 350°F. Lightly coat an 8-inch-square baking pan with nonstick cooking spray.

**2.** In a medium bowl, combine the flour, oil, and confectioners' sugar. It will be crumbly, so roll up your sleeves and get your hands dirty (wash them first, please). Work the mixture to create a uniform dough. Transfer the dough to the prepared baking pan. Firmly press it out to the corners of the pan to create a thin layer of crust, about ¼ inch thick. Bake for 8 minutes. It will still be soft to the touch and should still be white.

**3.** While the crust is baking, combine the lemon juice, milk, cane sugar, and vanilla in a small saucepot. In a separate small bowl, whisk together the water and cornstarch to create a slurry.

**4.** Bring the lemon mixture in the saucepot to a boil over medium heat, then reduce to a simmer. Slowly stir in the cornstarch slurry and continue cooking, stirring occasionally, for 3 to 5 minutes, until the mixture thickens up to the texture of a thin pudding.

**5.** Spread the lemon mixture over the top of the crust in the baking pan, cover, and refrigerate overnight to set. Cut into squares and sprinkle with confectioners' sugar. Serve chilled.

**OUTRAGEOUS ORANGE BARS:** Replace the lemon juice with ½ cup freshly squeezed orange juice (about 2 oranges).

**PERFECT PINEAPPLE BARS:** Replace the lemon juice with ½ cup fresh or canned pineapple juice.

**TIP:** *A great way to ensure easy removal of these lemon squares—or brownies or any type of flat bars—is to line the baking pan with parchment paper that overhangs the sides. After baking and cooling, use the overhanging parchment as "handles" to lift the bars right out onto a cutting board, ready to be cut into perfect squares.*

# Classic Vanilla Cupcakes with Buttercream Frosting

NF

**FOR THE CUPCAKES**

1¾ cups all-purpose flour

1 cup organic cane sugar

1 teaspoon baking powder

1 teaspoon baking soda

½ teaspoon sea salt

1 cup unsweetened soy or almond milk

½ cup canola oil

1 tablespoon apple cider vinegar

1 tablespoon vanilla extract

**FOR THE FROSTING**

½ cup vegan butter, at room temperature

½ cup vegetable shortening, at room temperature

1½ teaspoons vanilla extract

3½ cups organic confectioners' sugar

1 to 3 teaspoons unsweetened soy or almond milk, as needed

**MAKES 16 CUPCAKES • PREP TIME: 15 MINUTES • COOK TIME: 20 MINUTES**

If there is one thing I know, it's a vegan cupcake. I have traveled all over the United States and not once have I ever said no to a cupcake—not once. To my delight, I can't recall a time I have ever been disappointed, either. While some places love to get really inventive with their cupcakes, and I certainly celebrate that, I find immense joy in the simplicity of a classic vanilla cupcake with buttercream frosting. Feel free to jazz it up a touch with the variations or embrace the simplicity.

**1.** Preheat the oven to 350°F. Line 16 muffins cups (2 muffin tins) with cupcake liners.

**2.** *To make the cupcakes:* In a large bowl, whisk together the flour, cane sugar, baking powder, baking soda, and salt. In a medium bowl, mix together the milk, canola oil, vinegar, and vanilla. Pour the wet mixture into the dry mixture and mix until just combined.

**3.** Fill the cupcake liners two-thirds full with batter. Bake for 16 to 18 minutes, until a toothpick inserted in the center comes out clean. Remove from the oven and cool completely.

**4.** *To make the frosting:* While the cupcakes are baking and cooling, combine the butter, shortening, and vanilla in a large bowl. Cream the ingredients together with a hand or stand mixer until smooth. Add the confectioners' sugar, 1 cup at a time, and beat the mixture until it's fluffy. If the buttercream is too thick, add milk by the teaspoon until the desired consistency is reached.

**5.** When the cupcakes have cooled, frost them using a butter knife, if that's your style. If you are a little more advanced, get out that piping bag or small offset spatula.

## VARIATIONS

**LEMON CUPCAKE WITH CREAM-CHEESE FROSTING:** For the cupcake batter, replace the vanilla extract with 1 tablespoon lemon extract. For the frosting, replace the vegetable shortening with ½ cup vegan cream cheese. Garnish the tops of the frosted cupcakes with a little grated lemon zest, if desired.

**CLASSIC VANILLA CUPCAKE WITH CHOCOLATE BUTTERCREAM FROSTING:** My mother's favorite birthday cake combination is vanilla cake with chocolate frosting; I made this exact cupcake for her on her 70th birthday. Add ½ cup fair-trade unsweetened cocoa powder and 1 tablespoon unsweetened soy or almond milk to the frosting recipe for a chocolate delight.

**TIP:** *If you don't have a hand or stand mixer, you can make this frosting by hand with a big whisk. It will require some effort and won't be as fluffy, but it will still be delicious.*

# Salted Coconut–Almond Fudge

**GF** **SF**

¾ cup creamy almond butter

½ cup maple syrup

⅓ cup coconut oil, softened or melted

6 tablespoons fair-trade unsweetened cocoa powder

1 teaspoon coarse or flaked sea salt

MAKES 12 PIECES • PREP TIME: 5 MINUTES, PLUS 1 HOUR OR OVERNIGHT TO SET

Fudge reminds me of summers in northern Michigan when I was growing up. We would go for a day trip to Mackinaw Island and I would beg my mother to buy me all the fudge I could possibly eat in one day. This quick and easy recipe is an homage to those summer days and that delicious fudge.

**1.** Line a loaf pan with a double layer of plastic wrap. Place one layer horizontally in the pan with a generous amount of overhang, and the second layer vertically with a generous amount of overhang.

**2.** In a medium bowl, gently mix together the almond butter, maple syrup, and coconut oil until well combined and smooth. Add the cocoa powder and gently stir it into the mixture until well combined and creamy.

**3.** Pour the mixture into the prepared pan and sprinkle with the sea salt. Bring the overflowing edges of the plastic wrap over the top of the fudge to completely cover it. Place the pan in the freezer for at least 1 hour or overnight, until the fudge is firm.

**4.** Remove the pan from the freezer and lift the fudge out of the pan using the plastic-wrap overhangs to pull it out. Transfer to a cutting board and cut into 1-inch pieces.

## VARIATIONS

**ORANGE-CRANBERRY FUDGE:** Add ½ cup minced dried cranberries and 2 teaspoons grated orange zest to the batter before freezing. It's important to make the cranberry pieces small, so you don't have to chew large pieces of frozen cranberry when enjoying these delicious morsels.

**DOUBLE CHOCOLATE FUDGE CHIP:** If you like things extra chocolaty, add ½ cup mini vegan chocolate chips to the batter before freezing.

**TIP:** *When serving at gatherings, bring this fudge out in small batches as it will begin to melt within 30 minutes. You won't have to worry about it melting, though, because your guests will devour it. I promise! Refined or unrefined coconut oil, you ask? Whichever is most accessible, is my answer. The unrefined will have more of a coconut flavor, but both work.*

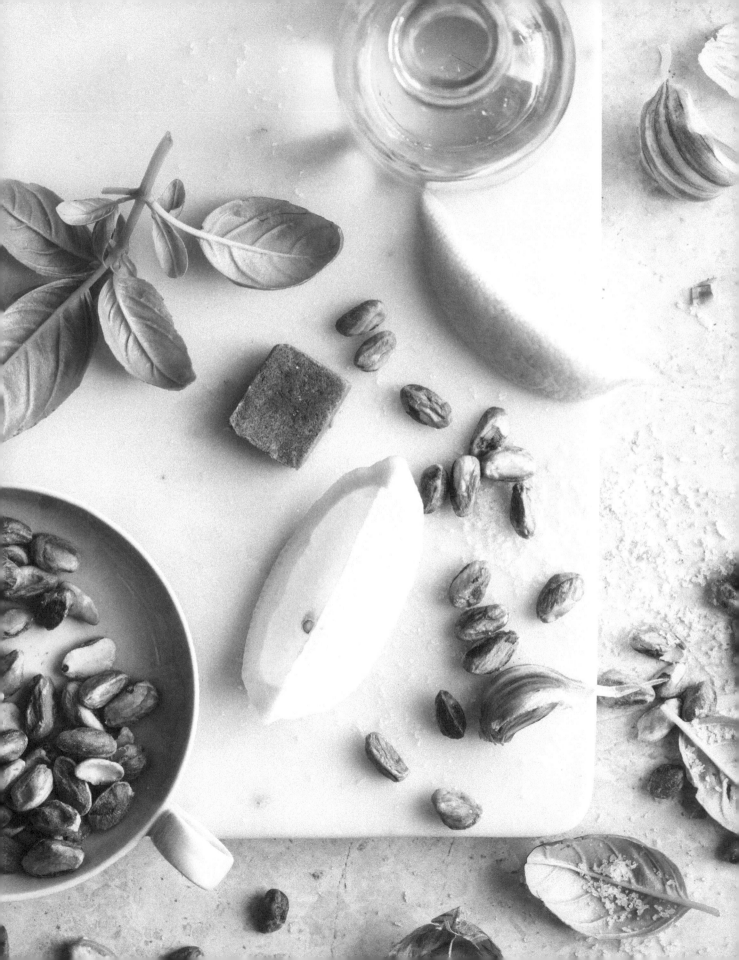

# CHAPTER 13

# Kitchen Staples

Supermarkets are starting to offer more items for vegan-curious consumers, and it is still a growing industry. But even with new products, many of us are being label conscious—as we should be. Just because something is vegan does not automatically mean it's good for you. For that reason, many people get into making some of their pantry staples from scratch. Beyond being label conscious, it's also fun and very rewarding when you are serving nachos to your friends with a vegan cheese sauce you made.

So far in this book I have rarely used what some might refer to as "special ingredients." But here in the staples chapter I do a 180 on this, for a couple of reasons. I think it's helpful to explore the marvels that are miso paste and nutritional yeast and, moreover, I would never try to pull off an easy cheese or pesto sauce without them. It's that simple. I wouldn't be doing you any favors by not mentioning these ingredients or putting them to use a bit in this book. "I really don't like nutritional yeast," said no one, ever. Try it, you'll see.

I have stumbled upon nutritional yeast and miso paste at very small, out-of-the-way grocery stores, but I've also been miffed and caused many a store manager to scratch their head when inquiring about these ingredients. In short, it's touch and go with finding these. But setting yourself up for success with a little online ordering never did anyone any harm. You could even kick it up a notch and do your neighborhood's like-minded shoppers a favor: If you can't find these ingredients in your store, talk to the store manager and request them. Look at the good you do!

# Taco Seasoning

3 tablespoons chili powder

2 teaspoons paprika

1 teaspoon dried oregano

1 teaspoon ground cumin

1 teaspoon ground coriander

1 teaspoon sea salt

1 teaspoon black pepper

½ teaspoon garlic powder

MAKES ¼ CUP • PREP TIME: 5 MINUTES • STORAGE: 6 MONTHS AT ROOM TEMPERATURE

Why is there taco seasoning in this book? Simple. Every time I attempt to buy taco seasoning, I get hung up on reading the label. There's usually some words ending in "strose" and lots starting with "dextro" and "mono," and I'm like, "Isn't this just a bunch of seasonings combined, y'all?" So I took it upon myself to make my own, because it makes me feel better. The recipe is easy, and a little goes a long way.

Combine all the ingredients in a container. Cover and shake like a maraca until well combined.

### VARIATIONS

**GARLICKY TACO SEASONING:** Add an additional 1 teaspoon garlic powder.

**CHIPOTLE TACO SEASONING:** Add ½ teaspoon chipotle powder.

**TIP:** *If you are someone who enjoys a weekly taco night, double up on this when you make it.*

# Green Goddess Dressing

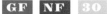 

1 avocado, peeled, pitted, and cubed

¾ cup water

¼ cup olive oil

Juice of ½ lime

1 tablespoon capers, drained

2 teaspoons soy sauce or
   gluten-free tamari

1 teaspoon garlic powder

2 pinches sea salt

¼ teaspoon black pepper

MAKES 1 ½ CUPS • PREP TIME: 5 MINUTES • STORAGE: 3 DAYS IN THE REFRIGERATOR

Green Goddess Dressing serves up a tangy punch of flavor that pairs so nicely with greens for a complete balance. If you are rushed for time, Annie's brand has been making a delicious vegan version of this dressing for years. If you go your own way and make this recipe, remember the best way to test your dressing is to dip in a piece of lettuce, taste, and season as desired from there.

Blend all the ingredients in a blender until smooth and creamy.

### VARIATIONS

**TAHINI GODDESS DRESSING:** Replace the avocado with ½ cup tahini.

**CASHEW GODDESS DRESSING:** Replace the avocado with ½ cup raw cashews (soaked overnight or boiled for 10 minutes, and drained).

**TIP:** *You see soy sauce or gluten-free tamari often in this book. Both are fantastic ingredients, thanks to their earthy, umami flavors, making them ideal for an all-purpose seasoning. The main difference between the two is that tamari has very little or no wheat.*

# Unhidden Valley Ranch Dressing

1 cup raw cashews, soaked overnight or boiled for 10 minutes, and drained

¾ cup water

1 tablespoon plus 1 teaspoon white vinegar

¾ teaspoon sea salt

½ teaspoon onion powder

½ teaspoon garlic powder

½ teaspoon dried or fresh parsley

¼ teaspoon black pepper

MAKES 2 CUPS • PREP TIME: 10 MINUTES • STORAGE: 5 DAYS IN THE REFRIGERATOR

Ranch attack! I find immense joy in pairing ranch dressing with just about anything, but I wasn't able to do that as a vegan until I went about creating my own. Those I have found in the markets are too tangy for me, and other recipes I've tried have either too many steps or unnecessary ingredients. This recipe is a straightforward, all-purpose dressing.

1. Blend the cashews, water, vinegar, salt, onion powder, and garlic powder in a blender until smooth, about 2 minutes.

2. Add the parsley and pepper. Pulse until well combined but you can still see specks of parsley and pepper.

### VARIATIONS

**BUFFALO RANCH:** Blend in 2 tablespoons hot sauce.

**NUT-FREE RANCH DRESSING:** Replace the cashews and water with 1 cup soft or silken tofu.

TIP: *You can adjust the thickness of this dressing by adding or subtracting water. Cashew bases thicken when in the refrigerator for a few hours.*

# Sour Cream

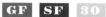

1 cup raw cashews, soaked overnight or boiled in water for 10 minutes, then drained

½ cup water

Juice of 1 lemon

2 teaspoons apple cider vinegar

¼ teaspoon sea salt

MAKES 1 ½ CUPS • PREP TIME: 10 MINUTES • STORAGE: 5 DAYS IN THE REFRIGERATOR

There is a brand of vegan sour cream that has been around for years called Better Than Sour Cream, made by Tofutti. Some people love it and others don't care for all the ingredients on the label. It comes down to personal choice. I use it in a pinch, but I prefer this super-simple and fast recipe for almost all my sour-cream needs.

Blend all the ingredients in a blender until smooth and creamy. Serve as is or refrigerate for 3 hours or overnight to thicken.

## VARIATIONS

**NUT-FREE SOUR CREAM:** Instead of the recipe above, chill a (13.5-ounce) can full-fat coconut milk overnight. Scoop out the solid cream and let it sit at room temperature for 15 minutes to soften slightly. Add the juice of ½ lemon, 2 teaspoons vinegar, and 1 teaspoon maple syrup to the cream. Mix with a whisk or fork until well combined. Serve immediately or refrigerate for 30 minutes to firm up.

**QUICK FRENCH ONION DIP:** Add 1 tablespoon dried minced onion, 1 ½ teaspoons garlic powder, 1 teaspoon onion powder, 1 teaspoon dried parsley, ½ teaspoon salt, and ¼ teaspoon black pepper to 1 cup Sour Cream. Mix until well combined. Serve immediately or refrigerate for 3 hours or overnight to firm up.

**TIP:** *This sour cream thickens considerably when left for a couple of days, but you can thin it out with some water if you wish. Or keep it thick.*

# Mayonnaise

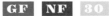

1 cup silken or soft tofu

Juice of ½ lemon

2 tablespoons olive oil

1 tablespoon Dijon mustard

½ teaspoon sea salt

MAKES 1 CUP • PREP TIME: 5 MINUTES • STORAGE: 1 WEEK IN THE REFRIGERATOR

Mayonnaise is an amazingly versatile staple—it can be used in so many recipes to give it that simple boost from dull to delicious. In the variations here I give you a couple of aiolis. Aioli originated from a Mediterranean sauce made of garlic and olive oil, but it became fashionable to call flavored mayonnaise "aioli" in the 1980s, and the trend has never stopped. Why shouldn't you be fashionable, too?

Combine all the ingredients in a blender and blend until smooth and creamy.

### VARIATIONS

**LEMON-THYME AIOLI:** In a medium bowl, mix together 1 cup mayo, the juice of ½ lemon, ¼ cup minced red onion, 2 teaspoons dried thyme, 1 pinch sea salt, and 1 pinch black pepper until well combined.

**GARLIC-SRIRACHA AIOLI:** In a medium bowl, mix together 1 cup mayo, 3 tablespoons sriracha sauce, and 1 teaspoon garlic powder until well combined.

**TIP:** *For a thicker mayonnaise, add ½ cup raw cashews (soaked overnight or boiled for 10 minutes, and drained) and blend until smooth. To keep it nut-free, use ½ cup rolled oats instead of cashews.*

# Easy Cheese Sauce

**GF** **30**

1½ cups cashews, soaked overnight or boiled for 10 minutes, and drained

1½ cups water

Juice of 1 lemon

1 tablespoon white miso paste

1 tablespoon tomato paste

¼ cup nutritional yeast

1 teaspoon onion powder

1 teaspoon salt

MAKES 3 CUPS • PREP TIME: 5 MINUTES • STORAGE: 5 DAYS IN THE REFRIGERATOR

I have been perfecting my cheese sauce since I first went vegan 10 years ago. It has taken on several forms from robust to mild, but I feel this one serves up the perfect balance. Refer to the easy variations below to spice up the party for numerous recipes or uses. My favorite things to use this on are pizza, nachos, and pasta.

Blend all the ingredients in a blender for 2 minutes, or until smooth and creamy.

## VARIATIONS

**QUICK QUESO, NACHO, OR MOZZARELLA CHEESE SAUCE:**
*Queso:* Stir in 1 (14-ounce) can diced tomatoes, drained, after blending.
*Nacho:* Add 1 tablespoon Taco Seasoning (page 219) during blending.
*Mozzarella:* Omit the tomato paste.

**NUT-FREE EASY CHEESE SAUCE:** Blend 1 (13.5-ounce) can full-fat coconut milk, ¼ cup nutritional yeast, 1 tablespoon white miso paste, 1 tablespoon cornstarch, ½ teaspoon garlic powder, ¼ teaspoon onion powder, ¼ teaspoon ground turmeric, and ½ teaspoon salt in a blender until well combined. Transfer to a saucepot and simmer, stirring frequently, for 3 to 5 minutes, until it thickens and sticks to the spoon when the spoon is lifted out of the pot.

**TIP:** *This sauce is on the thinner side, which is great for drizzling over nachos or pizza, but it will thicken up when heated and also when left in the refrigerator for 3 hours or overnight. It should be heated slowly in a saucepot over low heat, not in the microwave.*

# Fast Feta

**GF** **NF** 30

1 (14-ounce) block extra-firm tofu, drained and cut into ½-inch cubes

2 tablespoons olive oil

Juice of ½ lemon

1½ teaspoons Italian seasoning

1 teaspoon onion powder

1 teaspoon sea salt

½ teaspoon garlic powder

½ teaspoon black pepper

MAKES 2 CUPS • PREP TIME: 10 MINUTES • STORAGE: 5 DAYS IN THE REFRIGERATOR

This tofu feta comes together quickly and really hits the spot when you want that earthy, salty, tangy cheese flavor. Use it in recipes in this book or just make a batch to have on hand for your own favorite creations. I promise you it won't stick around long—sometimes I have it all by itself as a snack!

In a large bowl, toss together all the ingredients until the tofu is completely coated.

## VARIATIONS

**FAST TOFU RICOTTA:** Instead of cutting the tofu into cubes, crumble it into a bowl, add the remaining ingredients, and crumble it more until it starts to turn into a paste. Once it starts to reach this almost-pasty-yet-still-crumbly consistency, it is done. This can easily be achieved with your hands or by mashing the tofu up against the sides of the bowl with a spatula.

**CASHEW FETA:** Replace the tofu with 1½ cups roughly chopped raw cashews. Mix with the other ingredients and let marinate in a container in the refrigerator overnight.

**TIP:** *The feta can be served immediately. However, if made ahead of time and refrigerated for a few hours or overnight, the flavors combine and are considerably enhanced.*

# Pistachio Pesto

  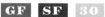

½ cup shelled lightly salted pistachios

½ cup low-sodium vegetable broth

¼ cup olive oil

Juice of ½ lemon

1 cup fresh basil leaves

2 garlic cloves, roughly chopped

¼ cup nutritional yeast

½ teaspoon sea salt

MAKES 1 CUP • PREP TIME: 10 MINUTES • STORAGE: 5 DAYS IN THE REFRIGERATOR

With this recipe you get the pesto both worlds. (See what I did there?) There are nuts in the main recipe, but I have also included a nut-free variation, because nobody should be without the opportunity to enjoy pesto. Whip this stuff up quickly in your blender and enjoy it however you enjoy pesto. I like it spread over crostini or tossed with pasta.

In a blender, blend all the ingredients until almost smooth. Some lumps and specks are okay for texture.

### VARIATIONS

**NUT-FREE AVOCADO PESTO:** Replace the pistachios with ½ avocado.

**PESTO WHITE BEAN HUMMUS:** In a large bowl, combine this recipe with 1 batch White Bean Hummus (page 43). Mix well to combine. Serve as a dip with crackers or vegetables.

**TIP:** *You can absolutely find shelled pistachios. Or you can shell them by hand, but add a few more minutes to the prep time here if you do. Keep your eyes open for the shelled ones and have them on hand to snack on, and to whip this up quick when you have that pesto craving.*

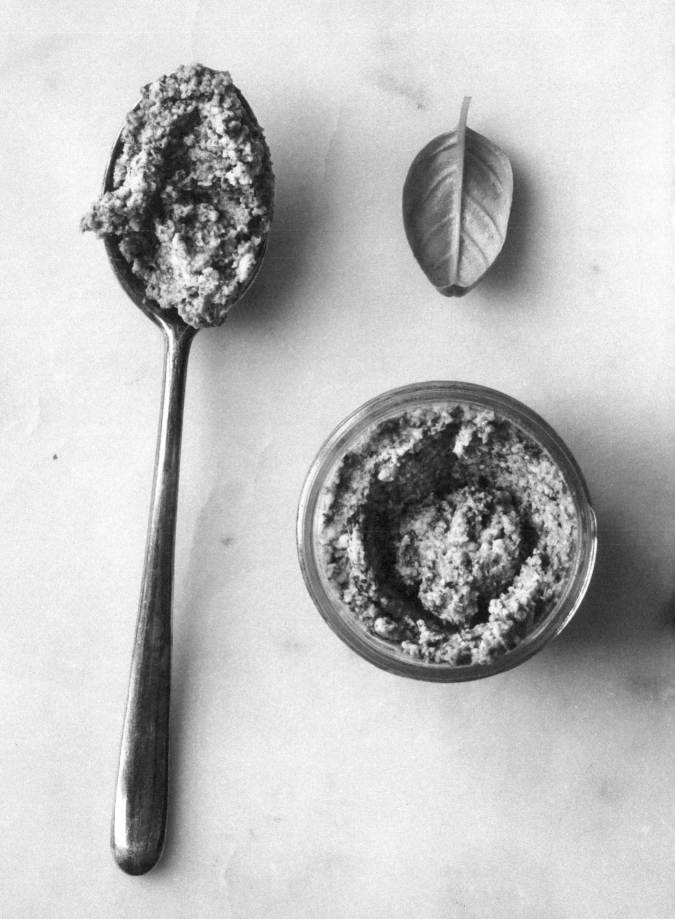

# Mushroom Gravy

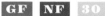 **GF** **NF** **30**

2 tablespoons olive oil

½ cup chopped onion

1 (8-ounce) package baby bella
  or white button mushrooms,
  stemmed and finely chopped

2 garlic cloves, minced

2 cups low-sodium vegetable
  broth, divided

1 tablespoon soy sauce or
  gluten-free tamari

½ teaspoon sea salt

½ teaspoon black pepper

2 tablespoons cornstarch

**MAKES 2 CUPS • PREP TIME: 10 MINUTES •
COOK TIME: 12 MINUTES • STORAGE: 1 WEEK IN THE
REFRIGERATOR**

The gravy train has arrived! I love gravy, as evidenced
in this book with Baked Fries and Gravy (page 131),
Swedish Chickpea Balls (page 60), and Country Baked
Cauliflower Steak (page 113). Here is the gravy you
need for those recipes, but I promise that you will find
a use for it above and beyond the options in this book.
Smother away . . .

**1.** Heat the oil in a large skillet over medium-high heat. Add
the onion and mushrooms and sauté for 3 to 5 minutes,
until soft and the mushrooms have reduced in size slightly.
Add the garlic and sauté for 1 additional minute, or
until fragrant.

**2.** Reduce the heat to medium and slowly stir in 1½ cups
of broth, soy sauce, salt, and pepper. Bring to a simmer.

**3.** In a small bowl, whisk the cornstarch into the remaining
½ cup broth to create a slurry. Slowly add the slurry to the
skillet and simmer until thickened, about 3 minutes, stirring
occasionally.

**4.** Serve as is or blend in a blender for a smooth gravy.

**TIP:** *Gravies are typically thickened with a roux, which
is a mixture of flour and fat, like oil or butter. I went the
cornstarch route for this book to keep it gluten-free,
but keep in mind that the Easy Country Sausage Gravy
variation will not be gluten-free because of the wheat
that is often used in vegan sausages.*

## VARIATIONS

**CREAMY DREAMY SWEDISH GRAVY:** In a large skillet, combine 1 cup unsweetened soy or almond milk, 1 tablespoon soy sauce or gluten-free tamari, 1 teaspoon apple cider vinegar, 1 teaspoon garlic powder, 1 teaspoon onion powder, ¼ teaspoon sea salt, and ¼ teaspoon black pepper. Bring to a boil over medium heat, then reduce to a simmer. Create a slurry by whisking 2 tablespoons cornstarch into 1 cup vegetable broth. Slowly add the slurry to the skillet and simmer until thickened, about 3 minutes, stirring occasionally.

**EASY COUNTRY SAUSAGE GRAVY:** In a large skillet, heat 2 tablespoons olive oil over medium heat. Sauté ½ cup onion and 2 vegan Italian sausage links, crumbled or chopped, for 3 minutes, or until the onion is soft. Add 2 garlic cloves, minced, and sauté for 1 additional minute, or until fragrant. Add 1 ½ cups unsweetened soy or almond milk, ½ teaspoon salt, ¼ teaspoon black pepper, and ¼ teaspoon chili powder. Bring to a simmer. Create a slurry by whisking 2 tablespoons cornstarch into ½ cup unsweetened soy or almond milk. Slowly add the slurry to the skillet and simmer until thickened, about 3 minutes, stirring occasionally.

# Walnut Parmesan

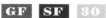

½ cup chopped walnuts
2 tablespoons nutritional yeast
1½ teaspoons organic cane sugar
½ teaspoon sea salt

MAKES ¾ CUP • PREP TIME: 5 MINUTES • STORAGE: 3 WEEKS IN THE REFRIGERATOR

If anyone ever tells you that you put too much Parmesan on your pasta, stop talking to them. You don't need that kind of negativity in your life. Instead, sit next to me and we will continue to create a variety of pasta-bilities and top them all with this nutty, cheesy concoction. *Buon appetito!*

**1.** Combine all the ingredients in a blender and pulse until well combined and the texture has become a fine meal. It will be necessary to stop the blender and toss the mixture around a few times inside the blender between pulses to make sure everything gets finely ground.

### VARIATIONS

**GARLIC WALNUT PARMESAN:** Add ½ teaspoon (or more, to taste) of garlic powder.

**NUT-FREE PARMESAN:** Replace the walnuts with ½ cup of hemp seeds.

**TIP:** *You can use raw almonds or cashews instead of the walnuts, if you want. The final taste will be slightly different but just as delicious. If you have a food processor, use that instead of a blender. The grinding will be a little easier.*

# Magnificent Marinara

1 tablespoon olive oil

3 garlic cloves, minced

1 (28-ounce) can diced tomatoes

1 tablespoon dried oregano

1 teaspoon dried basil

½ teaspoon sea salt, plus more
   if needed

**MAKES 3 ½ CUPS • PREP TIME: 5 MINUTES •
COOK TIME: 20 MINUTES • STORAGE: 1 WEEK IN THE
REFRIGERATOR**

Most of the marinara sauces found in the supermarket
are vegan, but nothing compares to the smell of marinara
cooking in the kitchen. It makes your dinner guests think
you have been slaving away all day, too. I promise this
recipe does not require that, but your friends don't need
to know.

**1.** Heat the oil in a large skillet over medium heat. Add the
garlic and sauté for 1 minute. Add the tomatoes with their
juice, oregano, basil, and salt. Stir until well combined.
Cover and simmer for 15 minutes.

**2.** Transfer 2 cups of the marinara, including juices and
tomatoes, to a blender. Blend until smooth. Return the
blended mixture back to the skillet and stir well to combine.
Taste and add more salt if desired.

### VARIATIONS

**ARRABBIATA:** Depending on how spicy you like things, add
¼ to ½ teaspoon red pepper flakes to the ingredients and
simmer as directed. Taste and adjust the seasoning to the
desired heat level.

**VODKA SAUCE:** Mix in ½ cup vodka with the tomatoes and
spices, then simmer as directed. Blend ½ cup raw cashews
(soaked overnight or boiled in water for 10 minutes, and
drained) with ½ cup water in a blender until smooth. Add
the cashew cream and an additional ¾ teaspoon sea salt
to the marinara after 15 minutes, and stir until the sauce
becomes pink.

**TIP:** *I prefer a saucier marinara, but if you prefer a chunkier
marinara, skip the blending step.*

# Basic BBQ Sauce

1 cup ketchup

1 tablespoon plus 1 teaspoon
    red wine vinegar

2 tablespoons dark-brown sugar

2 teaspoons paprika

½ teaspoon black pepper

¼ teaspoon sea salt

MAKES 2 CUPS • PREP TIME: 2 MINUTES • COOK TIME: 5 MINUTES
• STORAGE: 2 WEEKS IN THE REFRIGERATOR

My partner has a dipping-sauce infatuation. He will often order food at a restaurant not because he wants the actual food; he's after the variety of dipping sauces that come with the food. When faced with a choice, barbecue sauce is always his first request. I created this one to make sure I could throw something together for him when we don't have any store-bought barbecue on hand.

**1.** In a small saucepot, whisk together all the ingredients and bring to a simmer over medium heat. Cook for 3 minutes, or until the sugar has dissolved completely. Enjoy warm or chilled.

### VARIATIONS

**HONEY-FREE SWEET BBQ SAUCE:** Add 2 tablespoons agave or maple syrup and cook as directed.

**BOURBON BBQ SAUCE:** In a medium skillet, heat 1 tablespoon olive oil over medium heat. Add ½ cup chopped onion and sauté for 3 minutes, or until soft. Add ½ cup bourbon and cook it down until the liquid has reduced and the onion is still wet but the skillet has no more watery liquid, about 5 minutes. Add the ingredients as listed for Basic BBQ Sauce and cook as directed.

**TIP:** *You can adjust the sugar and paprika to reach the sweetness and heat you desire.*

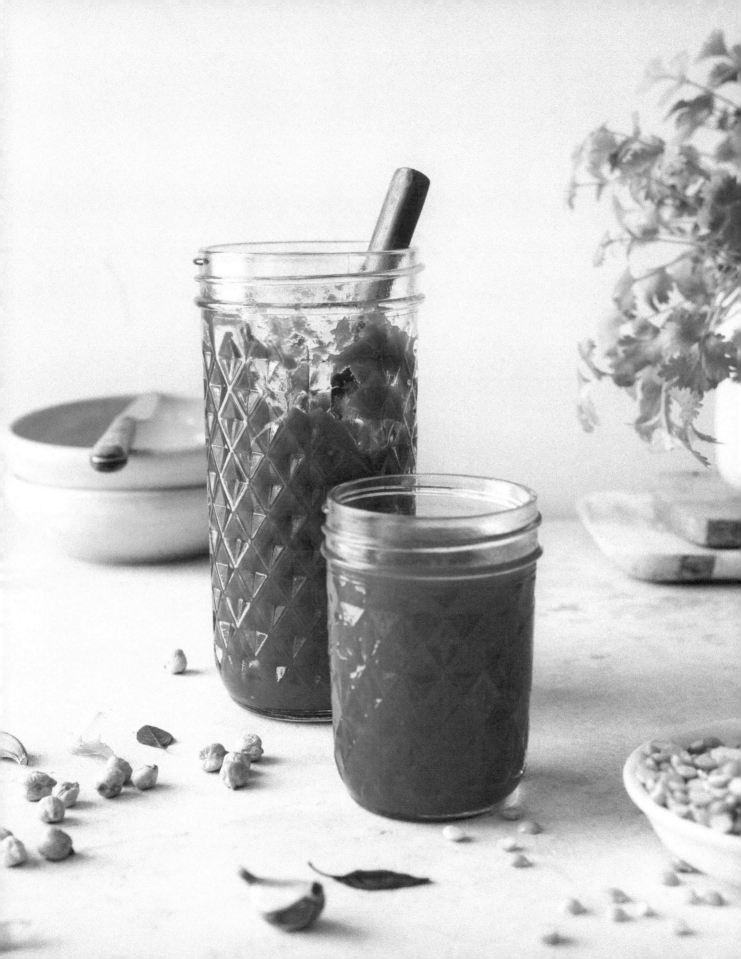

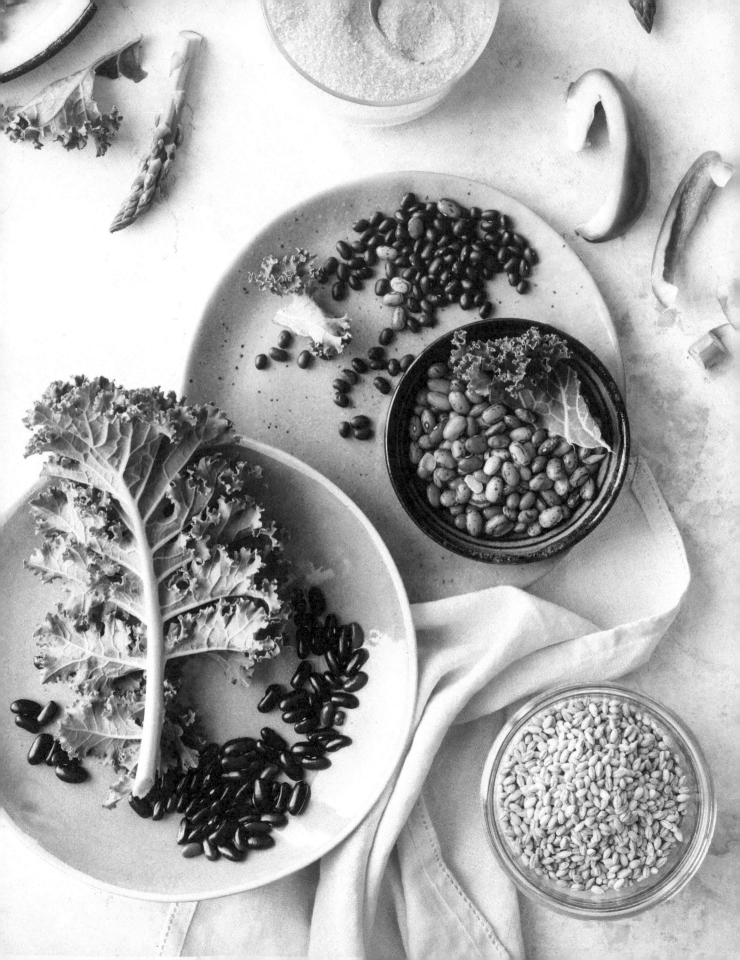

# Vegan Brands I Love

There have been plant-based brands kicking around since Wilson Phillips had their debut hit single "Hold On" in 1990. Some of them have suffered a fate similar to that of the Wilson Phillips musical catalogue (minus "Release Me" and "You're in Love," of course), while other brands continued to grow and have great success. Here are just a handful of tried-and-true brands I'm happy to recommend.

### Vegetable Meats
Field Roast
Tofurky
Sweet Earth
Gardein
Trader Joe's Soy Chorizo
The Herbivorous Butcher

### Cheese
Daiya
Miyoko's Creamery
Follow Your Heart
Parmela
Heidi Ho
The Herbivorous Butcher

### Mayonnaise
Follow Your Heart Vegenaise
Sir Kensington's Fabanaise
Just Mayo

### Marshmallows
Dandies

### Chocolate Chips
Enjoy Life

### Cookies
Just Cookie Dough
Alpendough
Enjoy Life
Lenny and Larry's Complete Cookie

### Dressings
Annie's Goddess Dressing
Daiya
Follow Your Heart

# Measurement and Conversion Charts

## VOLUME EQUIVALENTS (LIQUID)

| Standard | US Standard (ounces) | Metric (approximate) |
|---|---|---|
| 2 tablespoons | 1 fl. oz. | 30 mL |
| ¼ cup | 2 fl. oz. | 60 mL |
| ½ cup | 4 fl. oz. | 120 mL |
| 1 cup | 8 fl. oz. | 240 mL |
| 1½ cups | 12 fl. oz. | 355 mL |
| 2 cups or 1 pint | 16 fl. oz. | 475 mL |
| 4 cups or 1 quart | 32 fl. oz. | 1 L |
| 1 gallon | 128 fl. oz. | 4 L |

## OVEN TEMPERATURES

| Fahrenheit (F) | Celsius (C) (approximate) |
|---|---|
| 250° | 120° |
| 300° | 150° |
| 325° | 165° |
| 350° | 180° |
| 375° | 190° |
| 400° | 200° |
| 425° | 220° |
| 450° | 230° |

## VOLUME EQUIVALENTS (DRY)

| Standard | Metric (approximate) |
|---|---|
| ⅛ teaspoon | 0.5 mL |
| ¼ teaspoon | 1 mL |
| ½ teaspoon | 2 mL |
| ¾ teaspoon | 4 mL |
| 1 teaspoon | 5 mL |
| 1 tablespoon | 15 mL |
| ¼ cup | 59 mL |
| ⅓ cup | 79 mL |
| ½ cup | 118 mL |
| ⅔ cup | 156 mL |
| ¾ cup | 177 mL |
| 1 cup | 235 mL |
| 2 cups or 1 pint | 475 mL |
| 3 cups | 700 mL |
| 4 cups or 1 quart | 1 L |

## WEIGHT EQUIVALENTS

| Standard | Metric (approximate) |
|---|---|
| ½ ounce | 15 g |
| 1 ounce | 30 g |
| 2 ounces | 60 g |
| 4 ounces | 115 g |
| 8 ounces | 225 g |
| 12 ounces | 340 g |
| 16 ounces or 1 pound | 455 g |

# Recipe Index by Meal Type

## SWEETS

## THE PANTRY

# Recipe Index by Label

## 30 MINUTES OR FEWER RECIPES

# Index

# Acknowledgments

Drew Williams, without you this wouldn't be a reality. Thank you.

Melissa d'Arabian, your advice and support from the very beginning has been invaluable. Thank you for sharing your positive energy and expertise time and again. Chloe Coscarelli, you continue to inspire and amaze me. Your dedication motivates me to work harder than I ever have before. Thank you for everything.

Tim Eaker, Brad Snyder, Samantha Whetstone, Kelly Vieau, Justin Barnette, Meghan Rose, MK Flynt, Rachel Spadaro, Jennifer Hryciw, Kim Sosnoski, Cheryl Sosnoski, J. Elaine Marcos, Adam Peditto, Joanna Levin, Pamela Elizabeth, and Valerie Ramshur, your continued support, friendship, and encouragement make the journey I'm on worth every drop of blood, sweat, and tears. Thank you.

Thanks to Patrick Hurley, Dana Cohen, Michael Suchman, Nate Venet, Christine Pearson, Heather Suhr, Carmella Giardina, Diana Degarmo, Jona Favreau, Lacey McGarry, Karla Goodson, and Justin Leonard for lending a hand in testing recipes. Extra special thanks to LJ Steinig for not only tirelessly testing recipes down to the minute I turned the manuscript in, but for also shedding your beautiful light on this project.

Hugs and kisses to the faculty and staff at the Natural Gourmet Institute, the incomparable team at *VegNews Magazine* and the awesome folks at Field Roast Grain Meat for the continued support over the last few years!

My literary agent, Stacey Glick of Dystel, Goderich & Bourret, and publicist Penny Guyon of Firefly Media, thank you for seeing the pieces of the puzzle with me and believing in the big picture.

All the food used in recipe testing for this book made it to those who were in need, thanks to the contributions of A Well-Fed World, Neysha Vazquez, Stan Ponte, and John Metzner. Special thanks to Alex Caruso, who helped me get the food to the homeless every single week, several times in the rain. Your contribution of time and effort meant the world to me.

Bill and Dorothy Berloni, thank you for encouraging me to pursue my passions and for letting me be part of your family even as my work has taken me elsewhere.

Stacy Wagner-Kinnear and the team at Callisto Media, thank you for your fierce dedication to this project and for choosing me to collaborate with!

Ashley Madden, there is nobody else I would rather have in-depth conversations with about red bell peppers, onions, and lentils. Thank you for always being there for me.

To the countless chefs and business owners I worked with while filming the first two seasons of *The Vegan Roadie*, you inspired me, you encouraged me, and most importantly, you educated me. Thank you.

Mom, Dad, Sunshine, and Tyler, thank you for always believing in every crazy idea and adventure I have decided to pursue. Sometimes I have crashed; other times I have soared. Having a family that believes in me no matter what and understands the sacrifices it takes to create has generated a world of possibilities for me; I am forever grateful.

David Rossetti, it takes courage to taste test Caesar dressing at 7 a.m. Thank you for never hesitating when I needed your taste buds, for putting up with me blasting music to fuel my creative juices at all hours, and for helping me stay sane when there weren't enough hours in the day—and that kitchen just wasn't big enough! This book would not have been possible without you, but really, can we figure out how to add a 25th hour? I love you.

Finally, to every meat-and-potatoes-loving and "But I could never give up cheese"-declaring person out there . . . I totally get it. I was once there too. My life since going vegan has taught me many things, and I'm grateful to share some of them with you in this book. Who knows, maybe you will learn something too! No matter where you are on your journey, thank you for buying this book and giving plants a try.

Keep on cooking y'all, and remember, it's nice to be nice.

**DUSTIN**

# About the Author

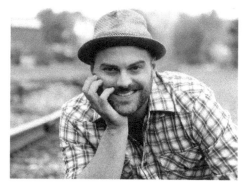

**Dustin Harder** is the host and creator of the original vegan travel culinary series *The Vegan Roadie*. When not on the road filming, Dustin is home in NYC serving clients as a personal plant-based chef and working with various restaurants in recipe development. Dustin worked alongside celebrity chef Chloe Coscarelli to develop her recipes for the fast casual chain By Chloe. Also an educator, Dustin teaches his Vegan Roadie Cooking Course at various venues around the United States and at the Natural Gourmet Institute in New York City, from which he is also a graduate. Having traveled over 110,000 miles around America in the last 10 years working with chefs of all levels, Dustin has seen and tasted the food that America wants and knows how to make it easy and accessible.

Facebook, Instagram, and Twitter: @TheVeganRoadie

CPSIA information can be obtained
at www.ICGtesting.com
Printed in the USA
LVHW05s1727091018
592727LV00001BA/1/P

9 781623 159269